The law of

Attraction

Freaking works!

The Inner-game to manifest

the skinny,

healthy,

vivacious version

of you with ease;

even after childbirth

•••

ISBN-10: 1530249775

ISBN-13: 978-1530249770

CONTENTS

Gratitude

and Dedication

I am extremely grateful to my Angels
Both physical and non-physical
Who continue to show up
On my journey
In countless ways,
Leaving deep marks;
Some camouflaged as scars,
But serve as lessons, wisdom and
reminders of my own brilliance,
uniqueness and radiance.

* * *

I dedicate this book to you,
my fellow Mom, Girlfriend, Sister,
or whoever is seeking to expand their consciousness--
unafraid to challenge certain past beliefs.
I honor and respect you for being open to embrace
the truth that lies within your soul: that **secret** and
sacred space flaming with Divine sparks and visions;
waiting for you to unlock the hidden treasures of your
ever-evolving Sacred Self...

* * *

Be **FREE** to harness the power of your desires.
FEEL free to embody boldness,
to choose the path of your manifestation
that **FEELS** magical.

***

Because, you know what?
There is something about your desire that is beyond
the solid matter of body & flesh:
It is a sound - the sound of Go(o)d music,
Asking to play through you.
Fall in love with 'That Sound'
Allow it ...
Be it...

With hope, it is
believable

With faith, it is
possible

With love, it is
absolutely magical

The story behind this

"LAW OF ATTRACTION

FREAKING WORKS"

book

Every journey reveals something NEW: a new way of looking at things and/or a new way of looking at ourselves. Thus even the 'destination' isn't just a place we arrive at, but a gateway leading to new adventures. Relax and enjoy the unfolding… It is after all, your saga…

There's absolutely no way I would be writing this book if my 'God'dess Self didn't hold my hands, literary...

Oh Therra, how dare you use the word Goddess? I've been asked that several times...

Oh, how dare any woman chooses to identify with anything less? I am not shy about owning my worth as a 'Goddess'.

Unlike what many have been made to believe, it is nothing mystical, it has nothing to do with equating myself to God or sounding grandiose; but a candid declaration infused with freedom, truth and love. The plain and simple truth is: *greater is the Spirit withIN me* than most of the wimpy made-up lies instigated by society to distort our identity, heighten fear, peer pressure, division, scarcity and mediocrity. Our identity is easily the most important thing, yet always at war – one day, fear is asking you to take her advice about Self-doubt and the next minute, faith is offering you a badge of honor; both vying for your identity...

But you know what? The moment you honor your worth and identity (as a Goddess) and choose faith, your purpose here on earth becomes rich with enthusiasm. I always ask: Which is better – to think highly of ourselves or to sit around and fill our minds with inferior depressing thoughts? Well, you probably know my answer...

I am FREE because my Spirit spans beyond my body and any flesh-related burden.

I am free to take the sacred journey into the deep; deep within my soul – where I encounter that confident Voice, the Great I AM, who speaks my authentic language, liberates my heart to love myself and others without condemnation. It Is the Voice that awakens my innate genius and creativity. It is the Source of my OVERFLOW: Inspiration, energy, magical ideas, spunk and... did I mention, an absolute pleasure to be with. Dwelling in the Kingdom of my Inner-Goddess, I find no reason to blame anyone, nothing to regret, no place for shame, but to joyfully float and evolve with the vision I hold.

When life on earth dares to overwhelm, when confusion lurks, I get sucked back into this 'Kingdom' to recharge and restore my peace, serenity and dignity. I encounter such EASE – the ease that only Truth brings! I meet grace and wisdom and allow strength-born-of-joy and boldness to activate my zeal, passion and tenacity for the journey ahead. In this 'Kingdom', I am my own Anti-Guilt Enhancer, thus I wear my wonderfully-made Goddess crown with smiles because I am able to ATTRACT beauty into all areas of my life.

I believe with all my heart that by virtue of having a 'womb', every woman is a Conceiver of dreams and a Life-giver who can ignite fire to bring light & life into dead situations.

Like pregnancy incubating a baby in the womb, and knows how to prepare the body when delivery is due, women are created to create. We're equipped to manifest magic. We just have to trust the process and learn to flow with ease – the Ease that only Truth brings. We need to allow every cell in our Being to experience the fullness of that ease. When other people, events or the mind goes on overdrive to distract, discourage, inflict pain or provoke anger, it doesn't diminish our worthiness!

Like a pregnant woman in labor, I have the options not to struggle and fight during childbirth. I can fight all I want, but I have the *option* not to. I have learned that in the course of co-creating my reality with the Divine Mind, the more intent I pour into relaxing and release tension, the easier it is for the life-force to steer miracles in my favor. In delight I am witnessing the magical unfolding of giving birth to dreams and very grateful for the effects on my body, my mind and lifestyle.

For a long time, I had been feeling an inclination to this topic (inner game of manifesting) so strong that ignoring it was not even an option. I was like a pregnant woman having cravings for something indescribable, a deep-deep connection that had my name imprinted all over it and was calling with piercing vibrant energy -- I Am That!!!!!!!

Thanks to that energy, this book was written virtually everywhere imaginable:

☆ in the bathtub,

☆ on the bathroom floor,

☆ the passenger's seat,

☆ the driver's seat,

☆ in restaurants,

☆ in churches,

☆ in the kitchen,

☆ at the park,

☆ at the bank,

☆ in the parking lot,

☆ in my living room,

☆ at the grocery store,

☆ out walking,

☆ while eating,

☆ while breastfeeding (thank God for Smartphones HAA!!),

☆ on my deck,

☆ doing house work,

☆ during baby's naptime,

☆ on the dance-floor (no kidding),

☆ in hotels,

☆ during road trips,

☆ on the plane,

☆ by the pool,

☆ on the beach,

☆ while pushing baby's stroller,

☆ while putting on make-up,

☆ in the wee-hours of the morning...

You name it... and my Inner-Goddess was there, always waiting for me to be the vessel. Did I mention during breastfeeding? (Oh yes, you can type with one finger on your iPhone while breastfeeding. Yeah, the secret is out — I bet I speak for several MOMS when I say we really do that. HAHAA!!!

The point is that inspiration was coming from virtually everywhere and everything. I guess that is where "God" IS, right? − *Everywhere and in everything.* − so be careful what or who you curse.

It may not always be the "devil", as we have been conditioned to believe.

There was this particular day I could not help but shout: *"My God, can you please slow down...* I was virtually having a conversation with this "flow-of-inspiration". As much as I enjoyed it, I needed to find ways to slow down in order to maintain my sanity and ensure safety, because on many occasions, I was driving on the highway or running too late to pull over on the side of the road and write down what was itching to be expressed through me. Yes, it was exactly that – 'an itch'. What I am saying is that inspiration was in constant flow. Looking back now with fresh perspective, I realize I should take that as a compliment because I recognize what that means: I AM (present tense) a willing and open vessel.

Other times in between writings, I would just stop, take deep breaths and burst out crying due to the overwhelming love I felt within me, around me, through me, pouring into the words I was writing and reflecting back to me the essence of my worthiness.

At times I would crack up laughing so hard, you would think I was in a tickle fest with an invisible friend (maybe I was). The smile-attacks were nonstop, 'YAY-attacks', 'YES-attacks', 'JOY-attacks', 'BAM-attacks', 'OMG-attacks', 'Ahh-HA-attacks', 'Oh, that-is-freaking-awesome-attacks', 'I-knew-it-attacks' were nonstop... It felt literary out of this world; *like the rays of light awakening my cells to dance the tune of Divine passion!*

This process of "channeling My Inner Goddess" or The Great I AM, has been surreal to say the least. It is so freeing and joyful. It has aligned me with my Truest friend: ME, using all the pieces of my soul as a gift to the world. The reality of flowing with the synergy of such inspiration has become an addiction of Heavenly proportions. Sometimes even the clueless acts and the frustrating twists and turns were the exact building blocks I needed. It is very reassuring when you can master yourself and instantly change your feeling of frustration to Relief because you are Connected. *The reality of witnessing the unfolding, even now, is by itself, a miracle.*

I love reading, and I love that reading is a form of research, which helps you accrue information into the magnificent database of the mind. It also informs your believes and depending on what you choose to be exposed to, challenges the status quo................ Now.That.Gives.Me.a.High!!!!!!!!

I fell in love with reading ever since I was a child, and later with journaling when I hit my teenage years. I always had a knack for sharing: In my primary school days, I lived in a small town at the foot of Mount Fako called Muea, in Cameroon. After school, I would gather kids in the neighborhood and establish a "classroom" in my family compound. All I needed were a few souls willing to be my students and God knows, I never lacked volunteers. Who didn't want to belong in a fun, energetic classroom with a teacher who was ready to confess your worthiness? I am very sure I exaggerate when I say I was always graceful with 'my students' but they seemed to enjoy the atmosphere because it kept on going... until we moved to a bigger city – Douala, the economic capital of Cameroon.

Even in a new town, it wasn't long before I found peers of similar interests, mostly made up of creative nut cases. HAA! I was involved in several activities but one of the most memorable was the part I played in writing and casting roles for a sitcom we thought would hit the TV screens in Cameroon... Don't you just love Dreamers? HAHAHA!!!

I think our crew just wanted to enlighten people about the possibility of living life in a "Different World" and spread the awareness that it is okay to give yourself permission to dream unusual dreams. At the tender age of 14 or 15years, we had the audacity to contact a wealthy entrepreneur named Mr. Enonchong, to sponsor what we considered a very brilliant venture. He was surprisingly impressed with our ideas and willing to collaborate; but before long, our cast members started dispersing into the wild wide world; travelling overseas to pursue bigger dreams of their own ..... Fast forward 20+ years, when social media really took on, I continued this habit of creating and sharing; really not knowing where it would lead but for the pure love of doing what has always felt natural to me. Later my attention saw the composing of blog posts as a good outlet. The more I shared my story, my life, my creations, the more questions I got from the audience. I would spend hours replying to the emails, texts, phone calls and facebook questions coming from women asking me to help them with weight loss, mindset tips, holistic health or wellness-related questions... then it took a life of its own - I literary woke up one day, observing the sequence of events and poofff, it suddenly dawned on me and I heard myself exclaim: *Holly-golly! The Universe is aligning everything to publish a book!!!*

I don't know how I just knew but I realized that everything has been purposefully aligned to share my experience and wisdom on this subject of embracing a holistic lifestyle, purely out of living my authenticity. And that is what living authentically has always done, at least for me – it shines truth into everything I pour my soul into, makes it seem effortless and opens doors of opportunities.

Honoring the call to enlighten others who are on a similar journey brought clarity of purpose. I concluded that the idea of a book makes total sense: _ It is intended to have greater impact with more coherence and continuity than scattered information entrenched in facebook or twitter updates, texts or emails. I could see that the instincts to take those little inspired steps, even when I was at the tender primary school age began to make fresh new sense. I could see that every event in my life had ideals that were morphing into messages of great value beyond Me. I could see that the hints in every stage, even my mistakes were meaningful.

Putting this book together is not only to enlighten those who are seeking RELIEF and RESULTS in the area of weight loss, but over-all WELLBEING, because it boils down to the relationship you have with your own Spirit, the Energy that drives you; the essence of life itself.

Wow! Now I am really fired up*!!!* This is why we should never disqualify our intuitive voice. This is why the energy we pour into any inspired-action even when it seems illogical is still magnetic and attracts a domino effect...

Now I honestly feel like shouting...

I feel like praising... I feel like flying...

I feel like creating! Oh, the word "Creating" makes me feel Sacred. Is it same for you?

Have you taken the time to examine how you feel when you create out of love, your inner-bliss? Do you ask yourself if you are operating out of fear or peer-pressure?

For me, creating FROM Love is magical. There is no struggle when I just allow my Inner Voice to BE The Dominant Voice. It makes me realize that everything, even blunders and periods of stalling can be Sacred if we don't punish ourselves.

Have you noticed your sacredness? Or do you punish yourself with fear-filled "what-ifs"?

Noticing my sacredness makes me feel boundless, nation-less, weightless, free to move in the direction of what is in harmony with my the object of my desire; and expect the greatest of my dreams to manifest; such as the possibility of becoming a serial Best Selling, Award-Winning Published Author, changing lives through my coaching workshops and beyond... Why not?

To close this section, I encourage you to accept that it is okay to give yourself permission to follow your joy, do what feels natural to you, dream up unusual dreams. It is okay to pave your way on this journey of Ascension expecting life-changing results; and because that requires internal growth, get an invisible trash bin for those thoughts that want you to pull your hair out in worries, justifying your lack.

We can all rise! There's so much more...

You are Divinity-personified.

Period + exclamation mark(!)

~Chapter One~

The Holy-Trinity In

You, In Me, In All

Embracing the whole

Total wellbeing is about being aware of your wholeness and living mindfully. It is owning victory on the inside before it ever shows up on the outside:

Your Soul knows it

and your heart feels it,

but your mind must accept it,

then ALLOW your body to express it.

Soul/spirit, mind and Body: It is common for people to approach weight loss as a physical phenomenon. Others ridicule it for glorifying vanity and some even downplay the health reasons for shedding pounds. Everyone is free to take a stance on this subject and that includes me. Personally, weight loss is a spiritual journey of healing, a journey of discovering many wonderful layers of Self, breaking barriers, elevating one's wellness standards by embracing a holistic approach and expanding in awareness by listening to your authentic voice of Truth.

As earlier mentioned, I have always loved pouring into others, inspire and encourage growth either through words, art or wellness awareness. The magical recipe about this particular project is that combining all the elements of the whole Being (spirit, mind and body) that make my heart sing with passionate melody is an explosive blend and a blueprint for an AAAAAAAHHH-MAZING outcome. I am very honored that YOU reading now, are getting the chunks and bites of my True

23

Soul creations. Can you hear my heart singing? I am so happy; not just for me, but for you as well, trusting that as you internalize these words, your Soul will sing the tune of your own UNIQUE choosing.

I am constantly being asked about weight loss tips and the logical part of me has the tendency to respond with the typical answers: *"If you eat this, or eat that, and eliminate this or that, you will shrink your thigh or waistline".* Nothing wrong with that approach but there is more to wellness than meal-plans. *Sometimes people want what you have, but don't really know the behind-the-scenes strings that are pushing, pulling and guiding you to succeed...* so I strongly believe the ideology in this book will play a huge role to shed some light into those "behind-the-scenes" matters that will give you the confidence to fully accept your worth and build you into a winner. This is why I am so eager and ready in halleluiah-mode to answer the questions that beautiful ladies have been asking with earnest desire to get results. But before I go any further I want to get this off my chest: Having a skinny, healthy, vivacious body is Not about food.

Oh No, she didn't.

Yes, I did... and let me say it again: *A skinny, healthy, vivacious body is not about food.*

Don't make food the focus.

It is about Self-mastery,

About your state of Being!

About your sense of Worth!

About your Spirit-Identification!

In Other words, *Your love-affair with you,*

Your inner Goddess!

It is believe more in what you are made of so that what you see on the outside, even the plate of food will not have control over you.

I challenge you to ask yourself this simple question: WHO do I choose to embody?

Over the years I have availed myself as a human guinea-pig ruling my life FROM a Wellness-Awareness standpoint, as opposed to disease-awareness, and you know what? My body has responded according to the specific Energy of my awareness – I noticed the times I was struggling with my identity, fretting about losing weight for pressure-induced reasons, the feeling of unworthiness took over me and the likelihood of sulking in self-pity was very high. With that I was faced with the reality of feeling lazy, stressed, bloated, drawn to wrong eating habits, remaining stagnant or regaining weight, and then getting frustrated that I wasn't seeing results fast enough. It would stay on that high level of actualizing until I released the tension from within. This proves that our bodies respond to the cues of our innermost state. Every time I made the decision to ease myself into practicing the principles discussed in this book, I experienced a shift, which got me back on track to flow in the direction of rapid results. I'm therefore a staunch believer that manifesting a great body, just like your ideal lifestyle, is the natural consequence of marinating what you want, instead of dwelling on what you don't want. If you desire a happy life, then pour kind seeds into soil of your intentions and take action out of love; not because you are forced to, but because you find pleasure in it. It's like being a cheerful rather than a disgruntled giver. A cheerful giver derives satisfaction from giving herself or others love and care; and that's what we will be discussing throughout:- seeing your desires through the eyes of Love, feeling worthy of living an authentic, guilt-free life.

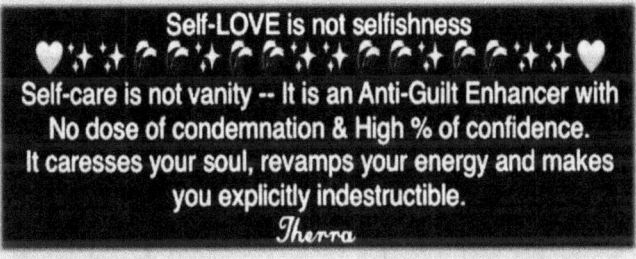

Self-LOVE is not selfishness
Self-care is not vanity -- It is an Anti-Guilt Enhancer with No dose of condemnation & High % of confidence. It caresses your soul, revamps your energy and makes you explicitly indestructible.
Therra

Thanks to the most frequently asked questions I get, coupled with what I hear from News sources in our society, I couldn't help observing that we, as a people have given very little attention and exposure to what actually goes on *behind-the-scenes* to attain and maintain that "dream-body". Frankly, how many times do you hear that your body and cells experience rebirth when you unleash your spiritual prowess? I have heard such cynical remarks to this assertion: *"doesn't that sound wishy-washy?"* And I understand...

Can you imagine a client at a physician's office being told that "the answer to your dream-body is to seek first the powers that lie deep within your soul"? I am laughing right now because I can see the face of that client turning into a blank stare, like: "Really, I paid you for this... to tell me I have the answer?!"

You hardly hear these principles in weight loss circles. From doctors to Fitness Trainers, we often hear of the emphasis placed on the physical effort, calories, sugar-free, cheese-free, fat-free, taste-free, pills, drugs, more pills; but not the spirit-identification of the person. No wonder so many Wellness seekers easily get overwhelmed because they have been conditioned to think *"if I 'WORK'-out hard, control my portions, restrict myself, take pills, I will get results."* Who can blame them? What do we usually see in the media? When famous good-looking people we admire advertise new trends in fitness, are we not bombarded by all the quick fixes aka 'miracle drugs' that melt away all your trouble areas?

But it is very obvious that when women make physical effort or restricting themselves their main focus, not to mention those wild New Year resolutions, they see little or no progress... and then what happens? Most of them give up! Heartbreaking isn't it? Where are those 'lose 7-pounds-in-7days' pills?

For a while I kept saying, oh, someone needs to speak up, or else this cycle of defeat will continue. I felt bad and tried to do my part; but how do you explain intrinsic details in a short text, email or facebook message? Well, let's just say... *This time, we are digging into the ROOT of the issues, so that we can have REAL manifestations;* from the inside-out. BAM!!!!!!!!!!!!!!!!!!

Okay, that's the only expression to accurately capture the truth of my excitement -- Bamm!!!

As I gear up to dive into the manifestation

ocean, revealing the essence of what really governs our wellbeing, let me tell you how I *KNOW* a thing or two about weight gain, weight loss and everything in between:

- *Clue number-one:* I am a **Mom**!!! Okay fine, that's my best clue. I have been pregnant many times; as in, many times. Wait, I mean, many many times - Most of my pregnancies ended in miscarriages. To be exact, I think seven miscarriages (I couldn't keep count after the fifth incident) and two stillborn episodes (at five and six months); and recently, a case of Diastasis Recti (abdominal split) after childbirth. All I am saying is that I understand what it is like for a woman's body to go through 'abuse' (for lack of better words), I understand the agony of shattered hopes, the suffering that can come from loss and ruin your focus, and if you're a Mom, I know that obligations can deplete your energy... But amidst all that, I KNOW for sure that our spiritual aptitude can conquer any obstacles.

- I must say that out of all that darkness, I have emerged a very bright soul and I still consider myself blessed-beyond-blessed with the three healthy living children I now have. I am not sharing details of my loss to invoke pity from you, but as fellow Moms, you know that getting pregnant so many times automatically comes with the green-light to shamelessly gain weight. Can I get an AMEN?!

- Besides, I am not one of those women who get pregnant and somehow manage to look 'un-pregnant' after delivery. Oh I wish!!! I am that Mama-bear who immediately triples her weight-gain numbers on the scale. As soon as my pregnancy is confirmed, you need to see me - I master my way to the fridge for midnight binges; even with blind-folds on. Can I get another Amen?! And I bet you know what I'm going to say next: *Who came up with that OBGYN's recommended range of weight gain, anyway?* I don't know who they use as Mom-models for that range of weight gain during pregnancy or what

31

those women eat (or don't eat), but for my size and height, I always exceed the entire spectrum of weight gained by the time I hit my second trimester.

- I remember one episode when I was pregnant with my second child and my husband bought me a gift certificate to a spa for massage. I walked into the spa and a worker, a nice gentleman saw me sitting in the lobby and I guess his mind added things up and speculated how far along I was, so he went ahead and prepared their massage package usually offered to third trimester Moms (Apparently there are varied techniques for massaging women based on trimester). When he came to usher me into the massage room, we struck a conversation and I proudly said "I am three months prego" He cleared this throat, jolted in confusion and tripped over his tongue trying to find the right words to apologize. Funny huh? But I am sure I'm not the only Mama whose pregnancy is known for giving misleading clues.
- I'm very familiar with the 'when-are-you-due'

questions, even after giving birth. You know those instances when you're seen in public without baby and an unsuspecting stranger asks when your baby is due? Yes, because my mummy-tummy would not fail to give it away... I'm seriously laughing out loud now!!

Oh well, I am very grateful for the experiences that my failed and successful pregnancies gave me; expanding not only my waistline but my consciousness. I learned that the light of my own Spirit could shatter any strongholds, turn darkness into clarity and amplify my purpose and identity – WHO I AM!!!!!

My gratitude therefore is not only for my living children, but for the many who didn't make it alive. I say that very reluctantly because even though they "didn't make it alive" they are very much part of the life I live now. Their story is MY story:

The last stillborn I had in 2010 was particularly devastating, yet remarkable. Baffled and shattered, my soul cried and questioned everything I was taught. As I walked the deep unknown path, seeking a way out of the pain and confusion of loss, I was also knocking down the walls erected around the meaning of loss. I soon found that peace was attainable in the midst of death, that losses are not always in vain. When I decided to let go of the physical loss and embrace the spiritual presence of my (dead) children, the sound of their voiceless voices and loving Energy of their collective consciousness lavished me with hope. That gave me tremendous courage to use my experience and wisdom gained as a portal through which another woman's fears could be lifted. But not knowing exactly how, or in what capacity to go about that, I simply decided to go with the impulses of my Inner guidance and I have been navigating this path since. How can such guidance be flawed?

They are part of what 'formed' and informed me of the ever-evolving woman I confidently call a GODDESS; without fear of being misunderstood. With this knowing, I take Gratitude very seriously and I see Faith for what it IS - It holds the secret of creating and manifesting: Faith is that fairy God-mother you want to have as you set out on your own transformation journey because every day, every hour, you are sure to unveil new truths about you that your old beliefs will wrestle with. Faith will remind you that you can shine with confident bliss even in the jungle of conflicting opinions. Faith will keep opening your mind, to observe the unfolding without looking back on the old bondage-conditioning, but trusting that what you desire is valid and sure to bloom.

~Chapter two~

With cool, calm

confidence, create.

From the unseen

"For me, I'm not going to be okay with just winning. I would love to break records…"

~Usain Bolt

Hello Life-giver/ record-breaker/ Winner!

I woke up today, a beautiful winter morning to a freezing cold weather in the mid-west, which is nothing strange around this time of the year. But the "tropical" kid in me is very thankful that it is warm and cozy inside the home of my in-laws, the place we usually bring the kids to spend quality time with their grandparents. Everyone is already awake, probably done eating breakfast, and occupying themselves with the many distractions that suit their soul and agenda. I personally adore these trips (especially in this particular location) because it feeds my soul on so many levels. When I am away from my own household routines, I have no specific schedule to adhere to, and this particular place which I lovingly call my "Retreat Abode" provides a welcoming, enriching, comforting atmosphere to relax, recharge, and do whatever... One of the "whatevers" I felt like doing was to stand in front of the mirror, look at myself in the eyes, smile and say: I Am Love and I can only Be Love and loved; that is why I see Love and that is why I love You..." and then I took a Selfie.

In the background is a beautiful armoire and a decorative piece that spells out the Word "Pray". It is a gift I got for my mother-in-law a few years ago and she chose this room for the décor because it goes well with the overall style and theme. Looking at the Selfie I took on my iPhone, the word "Pray" keeps demanding my attention and my Inner-Goddess did not hesitate to spew out these words: *My intention is not to 'pray' forth anything, because My Source withholds nothing from me. I always create with passionate smiles intoxicated by confidence because I am guided by Love; not by fear. Even fear is a type of fuel I use to accelerate... I was born with courage, with dreams and wings; and those with wings don't crawl, they fly. Those with wings don't linger in dirt, they soar. Those with wings don't look Up, but see FROM above. I Am my own answered prayer!*

Wherever you are in your journey, know that you are your answer. When you plant the seed of your desire, only you can nurture or destroy it because what you think about You becomes your harvest. Regardless of where you are, *LIFT yourself up, first with your mind:* There is always another door; unlock it.

There's always another height; Reach for it. There's always another level; Attain it.

There's always another portal; go through it.

Why?? Well, duh..... Because you can!!!

Embracing your 'Can-Do' Spirit puts your mind in ONE accord with your body, to break barriers and see the answered prayers rush to your reality. Usain Bolt, the Olympic Athlete obviously embodies that spirit when he says here: *"For me, ... I would love to break records..."* That, right there is someone who knows the power of his unlimited nature. It is FROM this position of personal power that he speaks with the confidence of a record breaker because he has learned that his body cannot go where his mind hasn't been. Speaking this way might intimidate some people, or can be mistaken for arrogance but it IS his authentic Voice. Like Bolt, all we need is to harness the courage to declare it and live it out.

Do you feel a lift? Elated? Encouraged? Reenergized? I ask because some people don't know how to lift themselves but seeing another awakened human helps to awaken their spirit. We are energies beyond bones and flesh and we're here on this planet as Angels for each other. Relax into that knowing and take a deep breath... Yes, breathe deeply, not tomorrow, not later, but NOW. It's the only time you have... Inhale.............and Exhale.

Once again, inhale..............and exhale. Relax and listen to what your Spirit has to say about your desire, then imagine your breakthrough. Suspend your doubts and boldly declare:

I AM a record breaker!!!

Now with cool, calm confidence, answer this question: *Are you ready and open to receive?*

*YES*_____

*Not sure:*_____

*No:*____

*** *** ***

I was first introduced to the Law of attraction and deliberate creation about fourteen (14) years ago after I read the book *"Manifest your Destiny" by Dr. Wayne Dyer.* It became a treasured tool after proving its effectiveness in a groundbreaking event in one major area in my life at the time. Since then, I don't put the book far from me for long intervals. I go back to it every now and then to refresh and to get deeper revelation of my own power as a *"spiritual being having a human experience"* as Wayne Dyer puts it. I understand that this concept can make some people scratch their heads because it is contrary to what society, customs, cultures, religion, families, media have been permeating into our psyche. We have been made to think more about the limitations of our flesh and bones, made to think like beggars in churches when we pray and to believe that in order to manifest our dream lifestyle, we have to ...wait for the word... hustle! Meaning you must suffer, hit hard, fight with others to take your position, etc. We are hardly taught that our desires can be accomplished by paying more attention to our bliss, pleasure, joy; the spirit that sees ease, appreciation, passion, excitement as our authentic and most dependable route. That is what really attracted me to the Law of Attraction in that it exposed my unseen world by pulling out the spirit-person and by personifying it, I gave value and respect to that part of me which is otherwise prone to suffer unfair neglect. Booyah!!!!!!!!!!!!

The beauty and delight of tasting the power of Universal Laws that govern our lives is that there are no limits. Everything is in our consciousness, awarness or the spirit-person; thus abundant in nature, free for all and flows *with* your internal rhythm. What does that mean for you? If you vibrate lovingly in alignment with what you consider your bliss: what is in harmony with your dreams, what is in one accord with how God, Your Source of Love sees you, your confidence in the outcome will make the process of giving birth to your manifestation much more pleasurable; hence seemingly easy. Your Inner-genius (God) whom you rely on, wants you to know that for every vision you hold about your life, there is also a way provided to achieve it. And you will know from your feelings if you are resisting your own Truth or when you are in agreement with it. With conviction, you don't have to force anything to happen because you can't force what is already yours for sure. Your Inner-Being delights in exciting you to bring about your creations with graceful ease.

Huh, ease?

Yes, I meant every word. I will explain later in the chapters, but manifesting changes in life using the Law of attraction is not new or some 'fad' trying to re-invent the wheel of spiritual laws. It has been producing amazing results in people's situations all over the globe for centuries. People whose situations were once labeled complicated, obscure, difficult and impossible have had victory. When I share the law of Attraction principles with

43

others, I often get asked why aren't the news media reporting such powerful and positive Truths? Are we so conditioned on negativity that we instinctively perpetrate the negative-oriented news and expect ills to happen to us? That begs the question only you can answer:

What channel are you choosing to tune in to?

Are you actively expecting information that ends up disempowering you? Are you seeking from the kingdom over-flowing with 'milk and honey" aka endless possibilities, or from the voices preaching vile, scarcity and evil? Are you believing the "evil" things you hear that drive you into fear-mode? Remember that Faith comes by hearing and Fear also comes by hearing. The only major difference is the One choosing what to tune into. You don't have to say you believe the positive stories about other people just for the heck of it. You have access to the same Universal abundance.

The ocean doesn't change color when Susannah or Emeka show up at the beach. It stays the same and offers the same depth, same waves, same potential for enjoyment. You may have to elevate your own expectancy to the point where it FEELS TRUE for you, so you can experience it in your life like the person you saw having a blast fetching water, swimming, laughing in that same ocean.

If you have desires of your own, and you believe you deserve to manifest a healthy balanced life, you can position yourself to reap from the bountiful Universe. By design, the Universe is here for your good, to provide for you, to reflect back to you outside what you truly hold inside (as your truth). Don't be afraid to ask the Universe for abundance -- There is no shortage. Does a child wake up in the morning and is afraid to ask Mommy or Daddy for a bowl of breakfast cereal? That has never happened in my household, and I bet you'd find it strange, even cruel if I told you that I have padlocks on all my cabinets for the sole purpose of starving my children. Ridiculous isn't it?

Nobody does that to their children, so why do we think The Universe withholds good from you. Why then do we, as a society rush to accept scarcity as normal, and teach our children that they have to beg for their birthright?!?

When you treat yourself and your life with shortage mentality, you are assuming that God is purposefully going around putting padlocks on your prayers and withholding blessings from you. The time has come on this planet when you must learn to relax the walls between what your eyes see and the enormity of what your soul knows, only then will you discover a well of treasure in your Being. Tune in, in response to the vision hidden in your imagination – your spirit world, your womb of creation. Tune in! Tune in! *Tune in!*

Permission to create:

The one thing I can confidently say I have learned from practicing the Law of Attraction is that anyone who desires more out of life can give themselves permission to create and I mean___Anyone! Isn't that awesome? If you can imagine, that is your foundation from where you build your dreams before it ever shows up in your reality. It is done with an elevated sense of awareness and promise you can only get from the unseen realm of your spirit-person. Your imagination is your womb and your dream is your baby yet to be born. Trust your imagination, feel your 'baby' in it, embrace it, love it and feed it. If nurtured in a happy, healthy kind environment (your imagination), your 'baby' will attract forces that will contribute to her development and find its pathway to enter this physical world for all to see. Don't you think such a baby will enter this world and radiate a happy aura? And until that baby is contaminated with lies about its limitations, it will prove to be unafraid to shine in all authenticity. That's the sequence of you manifesting your desires in a nutshell. It is like the process of conception to childbirth. The beauty and wonder of engaging your spirit realm is to nurture your dream by feeling the bliss of your endless possibilities. This is a sure way of transforming your life to match your vision, but done with joy and ease. It doesn't involve the resistance of over-thinking, rather the calm confidence of believing and knowing that 'you know that you know' that because you imagined it, it is possible for you. We are all endowed with Divine power within us that can attract and bring about manifestations with ease. The keyword here is ease, yes *eeeeeeeeeeease*. I'll give you a minute to let that sink in...

Have you ever asked yourself: *If God Doesn't Struggle Why Should We?* If God doesn't worry about bills and sickness why should we? Some will argue that it is because we are humans inundated with barriers but I say we are also more than flesh and bones. Can we not choose to have fun/ play more with the ease of our spirit rather than struggle with the confines of the body? If all you see is fat, obese and sick and starts losing sleep over those details, how does that help?

I believe it is for such reasons that you

have attracted this book at such a time in your life; intended to guide you closer and closer to tune in to that 'channel' of your inner Goddess that makes you feel healed, makes your heart sing, smile, laugh, and put you at ease_____ And I dare say, not only will your waistline change but other areas of your life you choose to address.

If you wish to manifest your desires in the area of relationship, for instance, please tune in. You are a WHOLESOME Being!

▶▶ ▶▶ ▶▶I have a sweet story about the title of this book that may spark a smile in you: It was born out of a playful, exciting revelation. One day I was meditating and feeling so much joy and appreciation for my journey, my awareness, my purpose, my life... and how all the pieces of puzzle have been attracting coincidences when it suddenly occurred to me: "Holy Wow! This Law of Attraction thingy freakiiiiing works!!!"

As I uttered those words purely out of the exhilaration I was feeling at that moment, right then I knew the title of my book was born. I didn't plan it. I was just flowing with appreciation and the ease of that Spirit gave birth to my book title... instantly!

There are countless instances where I achieved a total rebirth and superb clarity purely by focusing on the essence of the spirit that puts me at EASE. It is a stark contradiction to over-thinking or worrying which instead bring confusion. Thus clearly, the more I tune in to feelings of Ease, the quicker my vibration clears and attracts life-changing ideas to flow into my manifestations. So rest assured sweet soul, The Law of attraction freaking works!!

What that means for you is that as you spend time practicing the techniques, your heart will become more aware about the 'coincidences', about hints from your Divine Mind, clues, timing and what pleases your soul and cells. The more you deepen this relationship with your Inner-Self, the more you will become an unstoppable force with innate power to realize your dream body and life. You don't have to take the hard way to bring 'light' to ignite a situation as we may have been taught to believe. It is by staying in the flow of noticing go(o)dness in all things and situations, like children, that you will feel awakened, energized, empowered, inspired to take action. It is okay for us adults to imagine the feeling of liveliness and excitement like a little boy in a Thomas-the-train store. Are you feeling the thrilled already? Doesn't that sound like a sweet deal?

The Source of goodness loves that you want life to be sweet, joyful and pleasant; of course! That is the nature and fruit of the Spirit. And Go(o)d really enjoys giving more good, so don't hold back when it comes to immersing yourself in feeling GOOD about yourself. Find reasons and make up excuses if you have to. YOU are worthy, but no one can make you feel worthy if you don't already give yourself the gift of owning your worthiness! Own it. It is your birthright.

The better you feel,
the better your life feels!

It is okay (and very natural) for you to desire healing, prosperity, growth of any kind. We are ever-evolving Beings, capable of changing ourselves and transforming lives. Who wants to be stagnant when we are made to be on this ever-improving platforms of discovering how happy we can feel, how peaceful we can feel, how excited we can feel, how grateful, energetic we can feel. When you desire to be fulfilled, your desire is valid because no one is born to be locked in one phase of life. Everyone experiences the ASK-phase. But when you ask, learn to relax your 'walls' of resistance and be open for the BELIEVE-phase to lead you into the RECEIVING-stage, where you can see and feel all likelihood of your wishes fulfilled. You do that by taking your focus away from what you think might go wrong or what is lacking, to feeling FREE and OPEN to possibilities. Blessings flow better when the vessel (you) remain open. There is virtually no gain in allowing yourself to feel burdened.

Most people say they want a meaningful, happy fulfilled life, yet they put up walls of resistance and fail to give attention to what the soul deeply feels about the outcome of a particular subject. But thank God - The Source of goodness never runs out of ways for your life to be flooded with fresh, tasty sweet ideas and ideals. But how open are you to allow the sweet communion of the spirit to marinate into your bones, become ONE with you, fill you with LIFE, until being fully ALIVE feels like second-nature?........ Now all this sweet talk about sweet ideas and the sweet lively fruits of the spirit is making me crave my honey-sesame-crusted Almonds. No kidding! You can tell I am fishing for reasons for my cells to feel good, right? So off I go... to grab a handful of Almonds and I'll meet you on the next chapter.

~Chapter Three~

YOU ARE ALREADY

ATTRACTING

& MANIFESTING, anyway

Yay! You made it this far! I am super charged that YOU have decided to continue this journey with me and I acknowledge your open heart and your courage to stand for something that lessens the degree to which we entertain limitations and struggle. *What particular MIRACLES are unfolding for you here, I don't know, but I just KNOW they will occur because I believe in miracles.*

I believe your strong desire is already attracting a healthier, happier version of you and you are getting something needed for the next level, and that's wonderful because we all need each other – – each other's strength, each other's skill, each other's eyes, each other's wisdom. As I offer my hand, my heart, my presence, I know my words are filling your own heart with Light as you lean in and soak in the idea that being joyful, self-loving, free and inspired means you're truly living. As necessary as air, words are powerful and go beyond any limited physical space; that's why

It feels GOOD,

It feels RIGHT,

It feels MAGICAL to share this intimate time with you. To me, it means you are also called to this amazing concept, you are breaking free and manifesting your desires.

Why do I say that? Well, because as far as I am concerned, nothing is a coincidence. The usage of the word 'coincidence' is just man's limited way of making logical sense of God's Divine appointments. Your Inner-Being is pulling you towards what you desire; and it's great when you're so aware of not letting in resistance. Resistance can sometimes seem to spring out of nowhere but it's usually from past experiences, built up fears, or the ego. I'm so thrilled that some of the key things this transformation journey will polish is first and foremost, our Self-Awareness, then sharpen our intentions and help us relax our 'walls' so that we 'laugh-at-the-sky' more and not be too cynical when 'coincidences' arise.

Nathaniel Branden said "The first step toward change is awareness and the second is acceptance."

How True! I don't know how this book got to YOU, weather YOU stumbled upon it, or found it somewhere and thought 'oh what an interesting topic to explore', or it came to YOU from another beautiful Soul... it doesn't matter. If YOU are reading it, and feeling zingy, you attracted its **essence** to yourself. Focus on the **essence of it** – what feelings do these words trigger IN you? – These are the invisible forces inside you that go with the flow of your asking/intentions. Our existence is run by these spiritual forces and the spiritual realm (inside you) is very much alive and determines your performance in the world. Have you ever wondered what all the hoopla is about gut-feelings? A gut feeling is not tangible, you can't touch it but it is a language of your intuition that 'speaks' to get you to act upon something or see it from a different perspective. It is an integral part of your life that has always been there from the day you were conceived. The day you made your appearance into this planet is not the day you existed. Our relationship with our Divine Source, is older than anything else we have been taught by institutions such as schools, government, media etc. But breaking free from the control of any of those established strongholds to think for yourself, follow your gut feelings and embrace the wholeness, richness and abundance of Who you are at the core takes courage.

Many ancient scriptures carry parables, hints and principles of the law of attraction that support this wonderful relationship our humans Self have with the Universal Mind of God. And if it soothes the nerves of anyone who could still be skeptical thinking this 'law of attraction thingy' is off-the-wacky-side of the fence, or just needs clarifications on the depth of the impact that spirit has on our actions, well let's keep on trucking…

As a man thinks, so shall he be. ~Proverbs 23:7
The kingdom of God is within you. ~Luke 17:21
Faith is the substance of things hoped for, the evidence of things not seen. ~Hebrew 11:1
It is the Spirit who gives life… The words that I speak to you are spirit, and they are life. ~John 6:63

For thousands of years, spiritual masters have been teaching similar things in many forms, languages and different mediums. I think we have come to a point in time when we are flooded with information, yet some people are still suffering from LSS (I made that up: *"Limited-Self Syndrome"*). I am not saying this with arrogance to belittle anyone, rather with a heart swelling with love to AWAKEN you into the awareness that you are ALWAYS attracting, always creating, always manifesting whether you admit it or not. Why?! Because by default, we are wonderfully wired with spiritual energies to live this life not to toil, sweat and die, but to enjoy playing the game of attracting, allowing and thus manifesting based on the "seeds" we sow in our consciousness.

What affects the quality of the fruits >> the outcome?

As long as a seed is sown, sprouting, growth and harvest are usually imminent. The world we live in may impose many challenges to impede your growth but that can be remedied by discovering and nurturing *new* layers of yourself, *new* beliefs and *new* answers that enlighten you. Maya Angelou said: *"Now that I know better, I do better."* Always strive for better. Instead of being ravaged by fear or anxiety when faced with issues, you could invest your energy into faithfully nurturing the part of your Being that has the natural drive for creativity and answers that feel effortless. Such effortlessness is not easy to embody without Self-love, Self-awareness, mastery and transformation. A transformed mind is an imaginative person who is always open to see beyond the façade – that person who would question what the established agents of the world fabricate, impose or spread as "truth" and make the concerted decision to cast deeper into their ocean of Enlightenment. This person knows that the law of attraction naturally empowers the Wellness seeker to fall in love with her Imagined-Self first (instead of swallowing a man-made pill) because falling in love with that internal part of you frees you from focusing so much on what the limited physique can do. Your Imagined-Self is unburdened, free-flowing, ready to go anywhere and do anything. I understand that this concept can bring amazing transformation in one person's heart *yet* sound like pukeey-the-clown to others, but at the very least, you are now in-the-know.

When you know better about your Spirit-Self, YOU tend to treat YOU with kindness. *Knowing thyself is a gift.*

Nothing happens by chance, really! There is a reason hidden somewhere in your current situation even as we speak; but it is still up to each individual to DECIDE (yeah big word) whether to allow the inner-creative-energy to penetrate you, nourish the 'soil' of your seed and affect its fruitfulness! It is quite an empowered feeling to wake up one day from sleeping with helplessness, shame, insecurity, indifference and realize

Wowza so, it is entirely up to ME:

to make the mental shift,

to make millions,

to look fabulous,

to fall in love with life,

to allow the goodness of my Spirit to saturate my flesh...???

Yes, you are right; It is entirely up to you to open your life up to be nurtured and flooded by good spirits, in order to ensure good harvest. That is the real meaning of communion: marinating spirit, mind and body to form a delicious holism. If your intention is set to living healthy and vivaciously, then the news gets even better in that your body's ability to transform into what you want is so much greater than most of us have been trained to believe. The moment you believe it is entirely up to you, it doesn't even matter what society defines you.

From my experience with coaching, I'd say the one area of struggle for most people regarding the certainty of their own transformation and wellbeing is that when they see others winning and thriving e.g. the case of amazing Athletes, while on the other hand, other people are just repeating the same-old-same-old cycles of defeat... What happens is that the observer often allows doubt to consume them. *And doubt has the power to direct one's energy towards comparing themselves with others.* This thought-pattern influences people to define others as more "exceptionally gifted" than they are. This is clearly the spirit of doubt attracting similar thoughts that feeds into their inferiority complex. That spirit of doubt makes excuses, knows how to cover up and justify why you should crawl back into your dark holes of *No-Progress*. But Doubt is the liar and the fastest way to sabotage your own progress is to lie to yourself. Is that what you really want to manifest? I believe you know the answer...

My eagerness to drill into your mind what I believe your soul already knows is driving me insanely-high... and now I just want to shout:

Do Not Let Fear, Doubts, Insecurity Ever, Ever,

Ever Stop YOU from believing in yourself...

They cannot bite;

They are TOOTHLESS.

Yeah, chew on that......................

YOU are a masterpiece

It is your birthright to fulfill

absolutely-positively what you dream.

It's your DIVINE right to live your life in

"*Abundance-Ville*",

And never stop to apologize for it.

YOU are a Goddess;

Get used to it.

Not in future,

But *NOW*.

Believe it,

BE'Live it,

Be'Love it

Be it.

~Chapter Four~

BELIEF SYSTEMS

That's just how I See "it"

"All fixed set patterns are incapable of adaptability or pliability. The truth is outside of all fixed patterns."

~Bruce Lee

During our time here on earth, we have been acquiring substantial basics of mind programming conditions from the day we opened our innocent infant eyes and stared into the faces of those who welcomed us on earth and vowed to care for our wellbeing. As we spent years building those relationships, constructing our world, we allowed certain things to be automatically true for us without questioning them. We have clouded our subconscious with beliefs, ideas, thoughts, opinions, judgments, labels, feelings, and convictions that either free us, serve us or trap us. There is power in every idea as there is spiritual operation happening in every idea at the root-level. The difference lies only in your analysis.

How you approach your daily life, be it nutritional habits or lifestyle activities, is based on what your conditioning is used to identifying with. How you react to anything, or the meaning you give it, is in accordance with your belief system. BELIEF is the component or ingredient that makes "it" (whatever "it" is) TRUE for you. You may recite prayers all day long but without believing the words that are coming out of your mouth, it nullifies the effect. Saying something doesn't make it real when your heart is conditioned differently. Your belief system must work in conjunction with what you say, to have any transformative power because your BELIEF is what allows your behavior to flow easily in the direction it so chooses.

Hello, ever heard of
Cause-and-Effect?

A Cause is something that makes something else happen and an Effect is what happens as a result of the cause. You don't just wake up one day to find you're unhealthy or overweight. Things become your reality because you BELIEVE them and your habits develop over time to support that belief. Let's take this familiar scenario: If you are someone who has nurtured a belief system that waking up an hour early to exercise is such a hard thing to do, regardless of your "head knowledge" about how wonderful it is for your muscles to be trained, you're more likely going to fish for excuses repeatedly to stay in bed and skip training because your BELIEF dictates your actions and rules over the decisions you make pertaining to your wellbeing and life. What then will become the obvious effect of letting this BELIEF guide you? -- A non-active lifestyle, untrained muscles and a body-shape you may not be proud to show off in a bikini. Okay fine, your body doesn't have to be like that of a bikini-hottie; No pressure, but the point is, whatever you allow to soak in your subconscious, embodies you and externalizes in a way that you or anyone cannot argue otherwise because *You are a walking billboard of your Belief System.*

Believing Is Seeing! Heck, KNOWING Is...

Michelangelo said that after looking at a piece of rough marble, that he envisioned the perfect result or model in his heart before he unleashed it: *"In every block of marble I see a statue as plain as though it stood before me, shaped and perfect in attitude and action. I have only to hew away the rough walls that imprison the lovely apparition to reveal it to the other eyes as mine see it."*

You are not Michelangelo but if you are interested in knowing how to allow the ideal you to shine through, be aware that you possess his essence, and that you too can envision yourself "*shaped and perfect in attitude and action.*" Why? because you have the 'ideal you' inside waiting to be carved out. All you have to do is "*to hew away the rough walls that imprison the lovely figure.*" But you must question yourself to detect if your belief system is holding that person from coming through. Is your belief system at the doorway spreading her hands wide to stop you from manifesting 'your ideal'? Can you harness the audacity to face the 'rough walls' of those beliefs that imprison you?

It is perfectly fine to admit that you may need a miracle; but even a miracle needs your permission. Your part in this process is to KNOW that you can do it, and then allow it... and you allow it by not resisting it.

- Before you can EXPECT a miracle, you must be PREPARED for one.
- Believe that it is your time to receive what is coming to you.
- Believe that you are worthy to receive what is

coming to you.

• Before you can experience transformation of any sort, you must AGREE within.

You make your miracle realistic by believing in it and KNOWING for certain that no one can stop you; but You! Knowing that your beliefs will manifest gives you the energy needed to get ready and make room in your life to shine. Believe me, you have permission to shine!!

* * *

We have established that your mental reality is reflected in your physical reality because *"as a man thinks, so shall he be."* Since your creations come as a result of subconscious impressions, thus feeling your 'ideal' as true will determine your creation. Once you start changing your impression and perception, it results in a change of how you create, how you express yourself and what you expect from Life.

Creation Has A Method Of Progression,

so it is imperative to take ownership of NOW and just start wherever you are. The present moment is ALL you have. If you start preparing NOW for what you want, if you make room and practice, practice, practice, as if it were already true, it will be easier for your subconscious mind to accept it as part of your system. This is the freedom you have. Such freedom gives you tremendous power to break thicker walls of limits that imprison you and hold back your inheritance. Own your freedom! Express your freedom, and only then, can you blossom. Freedom must be expressed otherwise it is still confined in bondage. There is a huge difference between understanding this concept mentally and really believing that it can come to pass. Believing makes anything possible... Yes, the possibilities alone won't manifest out of thin air until you give yourself a chance to cement them by your choices, decisions and habits; all influenced by beliefs.

71

The Meaning You Choose To Give "It":

So.... Are you saying someone's Belief System alone can alter their challenges into success?

Ohh Yes!!! It is that simple. Because believing is seeing, and seeing drives your body into action! Everyone has a belief system. If you are interested in knowing how to allow the ideal you to shine through, harness the power of your desires.

A friend of mine had migraine headaches and every evening after work, she would use the headache as a reason to skip exercise classes; which makes sense to many people. But at the same time, she would get up every morning and go to work because she believed that if she didn't show up, her absence from work would affect her vacation hours and she didn't want that to happen. You see, in spite of the fact that she has a valid reason to call in sick, she wanted to keep as many vacation hours, so her mind came up with reasons to get out of bed every day and go to her job, sit on a desk in front of a computer screen for eight hours and perform her employee duties. Even though she was dealing with great discomfort, her belief system supported her decision to sit there and work under those miserable circumstances. Her belief system made up a reward and her body had to comply. When you wake up in the morning in spite of a cold and go to your job, it is because you have an established system that says if you don't show up, you won't get paid or you may lose vacation hours.

What are you seeing with your mind when you look at your circumstances? What you believe will definitely dictate your choices. No one is without a belief system. This is something that is so implanted in our psyche we act without even thinking of the root. It is for this reason that people see a glass of water and think it's half-empty, while others say its half-full, and others are just so grateful for having water.

Your belief comes first before you see things you want happen in your life. If today you decide to start defining your challenges as stepping stones, and believe this concept to the core, you will CULTIVATE a mind-set of overcoming the obstacle you're currently faced with or will ever face... ... ... if you even see them as obstacles at all.

Keeping the topic of this book in context, I dare say if you're fat (excuse my frankness), you better start jumping for JOY because you are carrying around so much value, you have no idea. Let that sink in... ... ... When you eliminate the counter-belief that your fat reduces your value as a person, you send that message to your subconscious mind and your subconscious responds to your beliefs. That's how you get empowered or disempowered. Despite how society makes us feel about it, there is nothing wrong or right with you being fat, there is only the meaning you choose to give it that has power to weaken you or strengthen you. If you see your fat as an opportunity to do something different, and use your story as a booster for others, then it has served you and served a greater purpose. If you have been approaching it with low self esteem, then these insecure vibes get you trapped. If you are at that point, I am here to plead with you: don't get trapped in it anymore, free yourself, see it differently... You are more than anything that could entrap you!

Bonus: Ritual Days

Have you ever heard of Ritual days? It is a FUN mind-programming exercise where you give each day a unique theme, and just in case your old voices try to interfere with your NEW goals, your subconscious reminds you of the ritual you decided to uphold and honor on that day. Ritual days have helped me develop the habits that have propelled me into the "Promised Land" of fit, toned, happy, healthy successful Mom.

See, you cannot arrive at your PROMISED LAND unless you develop a Love-Affair between you and your daily habits. Habits are just very small consistent acts that lead to BIG accomplishments. So without much ado, this is how my typical "Ritual Day" goes:

First, I would say, make it FUN. Personally I have been practicing with ideas of labeling my days of the week according to what I intend to accomplish; for instance:

"Let's-cleanse-the-crap-Monday"

(smiles smiles)

Monday is considered by most people as the beginning of a new week. As I enter it, I go in with the mindset of cleansing from the inside-out, both spiritually and nutritionally. I choose foods that are easily digestible. I become more intentional about my thought-pattern. I use uplifting words to describe me, my space, my environment and my interaction with others. I let go of things that obstruct my growth and clarity. I do this because I BELIVE manifesting my desires would require me to undergo the process of cleansing, clearing, unclogging some jammed pipes; and I'm not just talking about bodily "pipes", you know what I mean?

Unclogging old pipes refers to certain beliefs I have held about myself that may be keeping me from my ideals. If I once held the belief that eating cream cheesecake is a way of "enjoying my life", I know better to choose a belief that says pineapple smoothie and snacking on dates will give my cells so much joy after all they are sweet, satisfying and easily digestible.

My purpose for sharing this (ritual day) practice is to help you find a path with less resistance -- first in your mind, so that you do not contradict your own desires. This provides a leeway to pour the truth of what you really want, such as affirming beliefs that affect the your lifestyle choices; in a practical way. Another "practical" way I choose to show kindness to myself: Every Friday evening is established as ME-time!!!

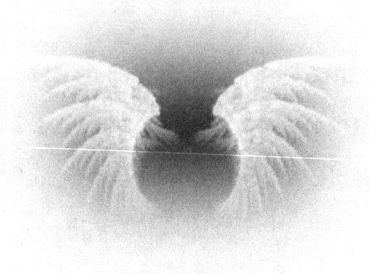

Your thoughts and beliefs are your wings.

Whatever you touch can soar.

You are an Earth Angel.

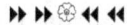

(Be)lieving is not something we conjure so that God

can make our desires happen.

"Be-live" is walking in the KNOWING that it IS

already created and has already happened,

so nothing or no one can stop it.

Hence "BE" and "LIVE" it.

When you are "be-living" it, you can experience it:

and things will unfold in ways that surprise *even you!*

~Chapter Five~

Just Say The Word

Declaring your truth

Living an intentional and purposeful life sometimes feels like the Art of re-installing new software.

But 'what software'?, You ask.

Just read on…

Remember that story in the bible where a Centurion met Jesus on the street asking him to heal one of his servants who was "lying paralyzed at home, fearfully tormented." During his interaction with Jesus, Jesus agreed that he will come and heal the servant. But the Centurion's response surprised even Jesus when he said don't bother coming to my house, for I don't think I'm worthy of your presence but just say the word, my servant will be healed. And even Jesus marveled at the Centurion's faith, that he turned to his followers and said Woah! This man's faith is so great and is rare, I am beyond impressed. And Jesus said to the centurion, "Go; it shall be done for you as you have believed." And the servant was healed that very moment.

Wow! Talk about EASE! This Centurion understands the idea of living life with ease. My West African people will call it *"No wahala",* that is, living without worries or living with ease. In other words why complicate things and make a whole ceremony out of healing? Why would you perform unnecessary rituals when you could just speak the Word? Sometimes we complicate things when we don't know that every INTENTIONAL Word we speak is a powerful spirit. This Centurion understands the idea of living life with ease. His first measure of the faith is that he didn't need any confirmation, as most of us would have. Normally, we would want to check all the nooks and crannies and confirmation-upon-confirmation.

We would want to first check the servant out, examine him, get the doctor's prescription, call friends, talk to co-workers and ask mother-in-law's opinion. And then go back and carefully watch that servant for several days, just to be sure that your faith is "working"…

Faith in an in-built EYE that sees beyond the physical – what a gift we have. Once you have "SEEN" yourself healed, or stronger, or richer, you don't have to keep worrying about what the outside situation looks like. There are in-built chemicals in our bodies that are made to respond positively when our hope rises and our faith leaps. So the inner-game of playing with your gifted-eyes will contribute a lot in making you feel vivacious. The lesson for me in this story is that we have to get in the habit of even *shocking* our Higher Self with what we say when stirred by our Great Faith. You will be surprised how your dreams and reality can quickly collide when you choose to align more with what your inner-eyes see than what other people tell you is factual. The Centurion did not have to see the servant showing any signs of improvement to belief that the Power-filled Words could go beyond the reality of the present moment to create his desired outcome in the future. Isn't it intriguing that through the exchange of words between the Centurion and his HIGHER POWER (represented by JESUS), the servant was healed at that very moment?

Very Intriguing!

Someone may be thinking: "Wait... We just discussed Gratitude in the previous chapter, talking about accepting and appreciating your present reality, and now we are making statements to go *beyond* the reality of the present? Help me understand because it sounds like you're encouraging people to be unrealistic. What does it mean to go *beyond*, anyway?"

I definitely understand your concern because I was once wearing those shoes of ambiguity about this concept. I agree that the idea of declaring things beyond your current reality may seem a little "out there" and a bit of a lump to swallow without fully chewing it, but if you give yourself a chance take a breather, you may be thrilled by how well it settles into your spirit, elevate your mood and sharpen your 'inner eyes'. Some people call this practice of using words that go "beyond-the-present-moment" **Affirmations** - where you choose to stay out of details of what is currently in your face, and concentrate on wisdom from your soul... because your soul sees beyond the confines of the flesh and knows more than you think. But let me clarify that there is no right or wrong way of making affirmations. Life is not meant for you to keep scores on what you get right or miss the mark. We humans have been taught to over-burden our lives with what is right, wrong, black, white, good, bad, ugly, etc. As long as your heart receives it in faith, affirm it!

What is the use of keeping something you don't believe in? It is like asking me to go to a gun-show and buy a gun when I don't believe in the hobby of shooting. It is like asking my friend to go buy a 5-bedroom house when she has chosen a lifestyle of travelling the world, pursuing her mission and has no problem owning just the bare essentials. Should I say then she has made a "wrong" decision by choosing a life living out of her luggage? No! But I have met quite a handful of people who spend so much energy condemning other people who made choices different from what was expected of them. Instead of spending energy condemning others, why not direct your energy towards affirming what you want to create in your life, and uphold only what you truly believe in?

You will digest life better, digest even food better, the deeper you allow yourself to be in sync with your inner-knowing. No one is taking scores, nor are you under a spell of judgments. We are always creating something anyway. Think about that and make up your mind to be in alignment with Creating, or fall in the trap of Reacting...

Reacting___or___Creating?

If you look closely, you'll realize that both words have exactly the same letters. I'll give you a moment to look again and discern what you just read. Isn't it ironic that something could be of the same caliber yet mean a world of difference when shuffled by the mind that is engaged in it? I've always been fascinated by the profundity and array of impact that "mindful shuffling" have in our lives. Most of us have been trained from childhood to react to situations after they occur, complain about circumstances, dwell upon our mistakes and condemn the ills of society, without realizing how much such toxicity it is contributing to repeating those same cycles of frustrations we cry about. As long as the mind is travelling on one side, summoning one-sided views (maybe based on what past experiences have handed you), don't be surprised if limitations sit comfortably in the living room of your existence. But some things can't stay the same, can they? In case you haven't realized it, *life is not static.*

Life is always in motion...

Move with it...

Flow with it...

There are always going to be heights to shoot for, to become better and efficient at prevailing over perceived limitations. I say "perceived limitations" because limits only appear big when we focus mostly on what our physical apparatus is observing. Yet nothing is static.

Everything is moving and subject to change.

Wow! I just read that again and mesmerize myself...

Everything is moving and subject to change.

Everything is moving and subject to change.

Change could come as easily as making a decision to implement life tools to tweak the mind to observe differently, then speak and walk according to the newly observed reality... all the, while getting used to the fresh, exciting ways of responding to situations.

Ask yourself: what if there is nothing to fear?

So instead of reacting to what you are faced with,

you can make a clear decision to let go of labeling the situation, and pour your energies into the creative process so that (with the nudge of your higher power) you can become a *Master at co-creating.* Affirming the things you desire before they occur is a big part of that creative process. Why? Because as you've learned from the story of the Centurion, which is very much part of your life, Words powered by clarity are impactful at overcoming limitations.

Express Your Intentions:

The act of affirming is like saying a prayer. The dilemma I have with the way we have been taught to approach prayer is that when we pray, we often do it like beggars; the "*Please God, look down on poor pitiful me and get me out of this pit*" syndrome. When we see ourselves as pitiful lacking authority, we identify as victims, thus denouncing our power. The pressure is heightened when circumstances put us at the border of a stiff place and an ocean; but even at that point, one thing we can do is to re-direct our focus and speak from another point of view. That's where Affirmations come in. The power of Affirming is that when you pray, express your gratitude for where you are AND what you are hoping for, as if it has already manifested; even if you don't see it, affirm it. I know it sounds wildly insensitive to suggest to someone who is in "poor-me" victim mode to look beyond that stressful moment. But, we need to speak more of that power IN us rather than the dreaded obstacles we *think* we are facing.

If this sounds to you like *"Pray Your Expectations, Not Your Pain"*, yes you hit the nail on the head. I don't know about you but it makes me feel better to speak to my perceived mountains with words that will illuminate my heart and improve my disposition, than words that seem to crush me every time I hear them. It is a shame that when people are experiencing health problems, there is always that temptation to drown into complaints and self-victimization. I am yet to find anyone soaked in self-pity who ever enjoyed being in that state. When you dwell in the state of self-pity, the problem only seems to persist and your wellbeing is more prone to be infected with that pitiful virus you wish you didn't experience.

The good news is that no one expects you to become the master of GREAT FAITH, believing in wellness and wonderment no matter what. You're not required to make a huge leap from a state of pity to a state of joy, just to prove or pretend that you "got this". But you can gradually talk yourself into feeling uplifted using helpful Words that can easily resonate with you and sound believable enough for you to stand firmly on them. There is a wonderful verse that stands out for me when it comes to the subject matter of self-edification using affirmations and you know me, I like to share when my heart is moved, so drum roll . . . . Ephesians 4:29: *"Do not let any unwholesome talk come out of your mouths, but only what is helpful for* **building up**, *according to the need of the moment, that it may impart grace unto the hearers."*

Okay, if you know me well, then you KNOW I am shoutingggggg!!! I can't help but scream BINGO!! You know why? Because I know with certainty that anyone who truly wants to set their intention on tapping into their potential, does so by *building up* progressively. In most cases, you can start afresh and feel anew and unshakable and inspired and rejuvenated. In other cases, your building up could mean giving up (cold turkey) on old habits, things and people that tear you down, while adopting a language that lifts the Spirit and matches the frequency of your destiny.

Point to note:

Building always starts with one brick, so where you are is just fine – start there!

~Chapter six~

"MAD COW"

Brain on steroids

I see challenges as FUEL for CHANGE,

needed to propel me to the next season of my life.

If you're honest, I bet you have asked this question: when my brain is running like a mad cow, how do I stop myself from speaking "unwholesome" talk?

Referencing a mad cow may sound funny but nothing fun about a brain that seems out of control. If you've lived long enough, you know what I mean when I say the brain essentially has a life of its own. It has the tendency to continually spew out memories of doom, images of guilt, scenes of shame. It is inclined to stir up the inner critic, the cynical voice in the head that never stops chatting. Even though I am actually convinced that no one is without the "mad cow", everyone has it within them to make an escape to bliss or at least, crawl to the brink of optimism. That is why I am jolted by hopes into believing that if we are willing, we can transform the negative self-talk into fuel for a better outcome. Like the Centurion in the story we just visited, we can choose to see challenges as fuel, needed to propel us to the next level of life.

If your next level is health related, you can transform using your inner-fuel. It may take going through several stops, detours of doubts and frustrations but with persistence, goodness and mercy shall follow you. A person standing outside on a sunny day seeing their shadow may conclude that life is gloom-n-doom if all they focus on is the darkness of the shadow BUT does it dismiss the ray of light that shines bright on them? What if you just turn your gaze to another angle and see what actually generated the shadow in the first place? Think about that. . . . . Your outlook changes everything about how you perceive yourself and your situation. If the "mad cow" is chatting you up on how dark and grim the shadows of your life appear, all it takes is a moment to shift your awareness to the ray of light that shines bright; and that energy is what gives you the drive to smack your obstacles down and wake up each day with the goal of moving towards the direction where your light guides you and your blissful results await you.

Henry Ford said:

"obstacles are those frightful things you see when

you take your eyes off your goals."

If that's the case, I say:

Affirmations are those promising things you say

when you turn your heart towards the Ray of Light.

What I am saying is, these shadows that appear in your life are a reminder of your light. Make it a point to insist on affirming the light. It is this minor shift that can catapult your vibration to higher positive levels and fuel your inner-Being to embrace challenges differently – as possibilities – as fuel – as game-changers.

When you stand facing giants such as your excess weight, you do NOT want to verbalize the things you don't desire to keep showing up in your life. You and I have spent quality time here reading about the Centurion, learning that your verbal language is just as important as your mental language because it is expressing what you feel and how you view your given situation, so before you rush to verbalize an old story about your life, give yourself space to ask: *Am I looking down on my shadows or looking at the ray of light?*

The V.I.P. (Very Important Personality) is listening:

Did it ever occur to you that someone very important in your life is always listening to you thinking, speaking, criticizing or passing judgments? Yes, you guessed right if you said the important person is YOU!!!!!!!!!!!!!!!!!!!! And you know what? Your mental "folder" stores these thoughts and when similar energies related to the spirit of what you think and believe hear you summoning these mental "family members", they follow the trail to that folder in your being. It obviously appears out of sight because it is all taking place on an energy level. The only person that can re-install NEW vocabulary into your brain library and change the old recorded beliefs is you.

If in-depth change does not occur, each time you press the 'ON' button on your mental computer, the "mad-cow" will automatically replay back to you what you have made the norm; and that's plain and simple truth about the Law of Attraction. Thus as a powerful Creator, it is critical to fix your vision on the shining light within YOU. Everywhere you go, you take your brain with you and it takes snapshots of thoughts that appear throughout your journey. As you practice turning your heart towards the rays of your light, even when the "mad cow" emerges, you have sharpened your intuitive sense to recognize that what seems to be a shadow is actually generated from light shining on you! And that right there, is your chance to experience something New and Fresh in your physical life. You are worthy of a new and fresh life each and every day. You are worthy of enjoying your time here on this earth!

~Chapter Seven~

How High Is Your

Mountain?

How HIGH IS your idea of 'Self'?

There is no mountain that exists outside of you. Everything you see outside reflects on how High or Low you place yourSELF. It always begins with YOU and ends with SELF. It always begins with YOU and ends with SELF.

The magnitude of your mountain is determined by YOU -- your idea of Self. In your quest for a healthy, happy or wealthy version of you, your altitude can only be attained by your outlook of Self. Your words, along with your beliefs can entrap your persona or can be very liberating. If your mountains of obstacles overwhelm you, it is because you are hearing yourself say:

Fear them!

Resist them!

Run away from them... And if you can't face them, grumble about them. It may then come as a sour pill when you tell someone plagued by crisis to implement something as easy as "speak to your Mountains."

You must be kidding! (Be ready for that question). Is this a game? They'll ask with cynicism.

My answer is, "Yes, it is a fun game of life." Our mouths were not just made to chew and eat but to affirm our dreams as well as bring down our walls of limitations. The words we speak about our problems can be the difference between stress and peace; which might be all you need to dig yourself out of sadness and be inspired into taking actions for your wellbeing. Always remember that you have this useful tool: Your Words; when fenced by mountains-of-issues trapping you in a web of fear. Your mouth is there for a wonderful purpose that goes beyond just speaking, to KNOWING in your heart that you have the power to free yourself from habits that lure you into captivity. This knowing is what gives you confidence to BE a force for good.

Jesus said unto them, because of your unbelief: for verily I say unto you, If ye have faith as a grain of mustard seed, ye shall SAY unto this mountain, Remove hence to yonder place; and it shall remove; and nothing shall be impossible unto you." In Matthew 17:20,

Your Higher Power, (represented by Jesus) is clearly not suggesting an absence of mountains, but the presence of faith and definitely the USE of Words. As long as you live on this earth, you are programmed in some way to see mountains or at least, think they are higher and tougher. Reliance on your faith allows you to access your authority, which you then use to SPEAK to your problem: "you are removed".

Any person with authority can hardly ever be

seen begging or asking others for permission. It is not just a quality you find in people in authority because they know they are powerful. They see themselves high up there in the ranks, high enough to command and expect results. You are that person! Yes you are that powerful person! You have rights over your body to command compliance and power over your life to command results in situations. Use your words wisely!

Facing a situation of weakness right now?

OPEN YOUR MOUTH!!!

You're not weak, you just think you are!

Feeling pity for your helplessness?

OPEN YOUR MOUTH!!!

You are never alone & helpless, you just think you are!

Exercise your authority, then Exercise your body!

Don't just pray and wish the 'mountainous weight' might be removed. Be more intentional and AFFIRM your desired outcome; especially in the midst of exercising. After all it is your life, your body, your abode... You have authority over your Kingdom, dear Goddess!

Embrace Paradox

Paradox: *A statement or proposition that, despite reasoning from acceptable premises, leads to a conclusion that seems logically unacceptable, or self-contradictory*

Paradox, with regards to weight loss is one tricky subject because of the irony involved. I see people struggling as they continue to identify, label themselves ***over-weight, plus-size or big boned,*** even after they have clearly stated that they would prefer a different outcome: skinny, lose extra pounds, build muscle, be fit and healthier. Anyone who understands and practices the law of attraction will confirm that they had to embrace paradox to win big with manifestations. When you start speaking from the *end,* as if what you desire is already manifested; watch your vibration shift - shedding the old identity that has been responsible for binding you, unleashing a happier you, moving you closer and closer to match the frequency of your outcome. You get elevated by your new beliefs to the altitude where you're so sure of your dream-size manifesting that doing anything that doesn't align with your vision seem ridiculous. When the knowledge that you are ABLE to close the gap between the present and the future excites you, that powerful force inspires you to take giant steps. The spirit of excitement makes giant steps less challenging, more exhilarating and makes you feel unstoppable.

I have been pregnant many times and obviously gained massive amount of weight - from 65-pounds to 70+pounds, but there was NEVER a time when I looked at myself in the mirror and said "gosh I'm fat." Ohh No Way! No freaking way! Such a thought is not even allowed to sit in my mind for five seconds. In fact five seconds sound like eternity when I even think of saying it loud. I know the power of thoughts and my Soul KNOWS that what appears in the mirror is subject to change because my idea of Self is more than what my eyes see. I remember the instances when people made remarks that my family members have weight issues; and they tried to connect it to my ability to shed my pregnancy weight using the 'family history' card. What they did not know is that MY Soul vibrates at a totally different frequency, nowhere near their opinion. What they say about me and their chosen labels stamped on my family doesn't ring true for me.

So how do I usually react or respond to similar outside opinions about me? I just shrug and laugh because I have an outstanding definition of Me. I know who I AM: Goddess of my life. Why not?!

- *Greater is the Truth within, than the outward illusion of scarcity and limitations.*

- *Greater is the Goddess within, than the superficial made-up fears and weaknesses.*

- *Greater is the GREAT I AM, than the opinions of others....* And I am willing to sound foolish (if at all I do) as I embrace paradox...

The Words You
Speak Are Life:

I think we have established by now that it is brilliant and necessary to incorporate Affirmations in the creative process. Without Affirmations, I don't know how I could survive the "mad-cow" and the "dis-Ease" of our racing thoughts. Having the knowledge that your Words have power is an arsenal. Your words, and the words of others have unseen energy. The energy is so impactful that it can attract similar energies to cause a compound-effect. I always tell my clients and mentees that I can destroy or enhance a child's life in a matter of a few years. There are certain things you can repeatedly say and with time, those repeated words they hear can form their identity and mindset. The words you speak or hear spoken to you can make you joyful or insecure, productive or depressed. In my case after childbirth, I could easily be discouraged if I didn't value myself and my opinion of ME so much. I truly understand when Jesus says in John 6:63

"The words that I speak unto you are spirit, and

they are life",

The more I delve into the spiritual realm to improve my understanding of how to attract splendor, the better I get at choosing my words. I am more aware of what I say and mean when I use certain words. There are words that accompany an icky-sticky distasteful vibration and meaning and I can feel it before I even open my mouth. And this applies to the words I allow myself to hear from others. When you bring up the topic of weight loss, people have some really messed-up ideologies about what to expect; and if you're not careful, you can view the entire process of losing weight as toiling and suffering. When you believe words like *"you're missing out on life if you don't consume ice-cream, cookies and soda"*, that alone can affect you on levels you don't even understand. When your spirit soaks up such words, your mind may not understand why you

105

experience low energy and often feel lazy to do what serves your goals. And even for those who put in some effort, for instance, to go to the gym may end up "rewarding" themselves with cake and cookies..... because at the core level, it is the twisted idea they have chosen to believe in.

Words drenched

In conviction:

As important a role that words play in manifesting, it is beneficial to know that the Universe doesn't just respond to mere empty words, but words that *match your vibration*, or what I call words with oomph or words with soul. I could say something like 'blah-zo-blah-zo' when I'm just goofing around with my kids and my vibration offers no strong spiritual force about what I just said and that would make it lifeless; thus insignificant in effecting any reality. I could say a rather cruel word to a friend with a playful disposition and when received with no hard feelings, we can both laugh about it, let it go, easily move on and stay happy.

But... Words that are drenched with truth AND CONVICTION are effectual on a whole new level. I remember chatting with my friend, a vegan, who told me that she sometimes gives meat-lovers a reality check on their weight and wellness goals by lecturing them about the feeding, processing and distribution of cows in America; in order for them to understand the effects of eating meat products. The way she usually describes it paints an extremely vivid picture for the listener to see the link between their stretched skin, bloating and the consumption of meat laden with chemicals and hormones. Listening to her got me so disgusted that I immediately changed my meat-eating habits. No kidding! I still feel nauseated just reminiscing on the details of our conversation. She was not even done telling me about this cow stuff when I stopped her in the middle of our conversation because I couldn't take the details in anymore. I was convinced and sold on taking my vegan lifestyle up a notch and since then I look at a piece of burger with caution and even disgust. Thank God grilled fish works scrumptiously for me and I can live satisfactorily ever-after with no meat.

My change in habit came as a result of re-evaluating my relationship with meat, which was definitely influenced by the information I heard from my trusted friend. I believed she was accurate so it affected my habit of eating meat. But is everyone going to stop eating meat the next day when they are exposed to this same information about cow treatment and processing? Maybe not; but if it sinks deep and resonates with you, you will definitely be affected.

Such is the power of convincing words!

~Chapter Eight~

Building The Bridge

Visualization + Faith + Trust:

Living my truth ... in my world

If you hide your deepest desires in the heart, even when your mind is acting the fool, that desire will find its way to birth... because the cry of your heart is so much more than the sighs (and noise) of your mind.

~Bernice Angoh

Your heart is an amazing magnetizing agent. As long as your Desires are hidden in your heart, even when your mind tries to trick you into thinking otherwise, TRUST in that hidden Truth, *that sacred and secret space*, and then project from there. You can use visualization to see your fulfilled desires based on what you believe in your heart; not what the chatters of the mind suggest.

Don't lie to yourself by pretending you don't want what you desire because that's against the truth in your heart (and only Truth prevails.) Being true to yourself is loving yourself. And get this:

"being yourself is the most radical but freeing

thing you can do."

The art of visualizing yourself well, powerful and whole, just like the beats of your heart is not selfish or anything you should feel guilty about. It is your divine right. Visualizing your desires fulfilled is just another way of asserting your faith. Acknowledging the truth (over and over) of what your heart knows is possible is a vernacular that Faith understands. And if Faith is the evidence of things not seen, I will dare say it is almost impossible for someone with complete faith in Divine power to speak against their heat's truth. If they do, that would be claiming defeat.

Defeat? De-what?

What does defeat even mean?

Well, let's not even go there because nobody is talking defeat here.

When I do my *Affirmations,* I find they are very effective when combined with *Visualization.* What you see with your spiritual eyes charges your faith-batteries to the point that you can confidently step up your game by taking great leaps forward to a life of Wellness; literary & figuratively. When I think that I want more of something to flow to me (from the unlimited Source), I would affirm something like:

YES, I see myself already slim.

YES, I see myself having more energy.

YES, I see myself with glowing skin.

YES, I am enjoying my radiant appearance.

Wouldn't it be nice if we took a moment each day to do this? Just say YES!!!

Anything you say YES to, you are affirming it into your consciousness. Once you are conscious of the body you are affirming and visualizing, while practicing the feeling of your healed body, slimmer waistline or energetic Self, *then you'll attract the spirit that creates such reality.* So every time you affirm what you really want, visualize it and do your best to feel the satisfaction of having it. Thus you are summoning the manifestation of it.

Knowing who you are, what you want, feeling it happening and acknowledging that you have what it takes, is also granting yourself permission to rise above anything that will hold you back, and particularly allowing the God(dess) within you to shine through you.

Sit for a minute and. . . . . .

Connect with that knowing.

Connect with that spirit.

Connect with that wisdom

Connect with that power.

Acknowledge it every day until you feel your inner-being embracing it, feeling enthusiastic about it, getting used to it and ultimately becoming one with it without judgment calls. How do you know you are becoming ONE with it? -- When your words accompany that feeling of knowing and make your every cell dance with joyful energy and vigor. That's how you know you are building your bridge to manifesting. In fact, you are already living in the embodiment of your desire because it is IN your heart; you just have to allow it.

Your heart knows it. – Allow it

Your heart can't fake it. – Allow it

Your heart doesn't force it. – Allow it

That is a basic principle of the Law of Attraction: Accepting the vision of your heart as a gift uniquely designed for you, using FAITH to see the evidence and allowing it by expressing your oneness with it.

WHAT IF PEOPLE THINK ... Before you even

complete that statement allow me to inject in here that nobody knows you better than YOU. So what if people think you're weird or crazy for affirming things that are not obvious?! I have experience in this area I can even write a book about it... wait... I AM WRITING a book about it. Haha! Well, maybe other people just need to loosen up or join you in the crazy club; if not, that shouldn't even be your business. What others think should have no bearing on what you establish in your life. Positive people tend to achieve immense results enhancing their wellbeing because they are ruled by the *heart* and abide by principles that others initially think are crazy/ out-there/ different from the norm. Learn to put a question-mark where it ought to be - Why must someone else's outlook on life ruin your desire to move in the direction of your bliss?

I personally know people who worry so much about what others think that there is constant resistance in their decision-making process. They cannot fully express the joy of what they dream, which holds them back, causes stress and affects their health. And such is the cycle you want to emulate? All I Know is that life is energy and energy is always moving in the direction you choose. You have the power to re-invent yourself anytime and express your goodness. Nobody has the power to stress you out until you allow them to take the position of power in your life where their discouragements affects you to the degree of slowing down your progress.

- *Only YOU know what you want;* Just say YES.

- *Acknowledge your faith in every situation.*

- *Don't worry about what others think or say.*

- *Be confident that your miracle lies within you.*

- *Your miracle is waiting to be expressed.* **Affirm it.**

- *Open Your Mouth and follow your bliss!*

Make it exciting:

If you are one of those who have been buried in defeating thoughts for so long that you still think this affirmation and visualization doesn't hold much grounds for you, here are some suggestions:

- *Your affirmations should be exciting and heartwarming that they stir your Inner-Being in a remarkable way. The good news is that once the words stick in there, nothing can stop you because at that level of the subconscious, it influences your behavior. This is why your affirmations are not to be practiced with lackluster and aloof attitude.*

- *Wrap your mind around the concept that Affirmations are not just words you throw around.*

Words affect how you feel and act. So don't be cynical because the spirit of pessimism will block its effectiveness.

- *You must be a devoted Monk to your dreams; someone who feels truly committed to listen to the heart's cry -- It is an authentic and genuine act practiced with heart and willingness.*

- *JOY is a component you surely want to add to this mixture to get the full flavor of benefits because joy is your strength.*

- *You are toning your spirit muscles, so don't give up before you enjoy the best part – flaunting the results.*

Remember you are always attracting by default, but now that you are aware of the law that attracts energies of possibilities, your game has to involve more instinctive fun and easygoing tactics to transform you inside-out.

117

~Chapter Nine~

HIGH & LIFTED UP

Christ Consciousness

The most valuable skill or talent that you could ever

develop is that of directing your thoughts towards

what you want. ~Abraham-Hicks

To live a balanced life of abundance, you have to be aware that the Spirit living in you is high and lifted up! In the spiritual community, it is often referred to as "Christ Consciousness." This isn't something you strive to achieve, but a gift you receive in your Spirit. Receiving the gift of Christ consciousness is not rocket science – it is just a matter of removing your focus away from things that bind you in stressful limits to things that make you feel limitless. A Christ Consciousness doesn't see a problem and gets entangled in the stress of it, rather seizes the opportunity to treat it as a precious commodity - polish it, nourish it and make it flourish.

The absence of Christ Consciousness puts one is a position rooted in fear and lack; which gives birth to unhealthy habits that breed stress. A guaranteed effect of stress is that it contaminates your attitude as it slowly sucks life and growth out of your being. I don't belief that just because we inhabit this earth, our lives are supposed to be seriously wrapped around the concerns of this earth, but that's what most people do... or have been told. It is true that we will get hit by darts of issues that can push us out of comfort but having Christ Consciousness swiftly comes to the rescue.

We are already created and innately gifted to perceive things from a view that is high and lifted up. Does this mean we ought to ignore our earth issues? No, it is not about ignoring, but we know better than to get entangled in the details that drain us; and that is what I am saying here. You have to learn how to command the Universe from a place of power. Your human side may need to repeatedly practice this for a while in your mind how to tell the "genie", your subconscious to: *"Do this with me"… "Change my outlook to that!"*. You don't have to be forceful, because that is a form of weakness, but with loving authority, assert your power.

I have a game I call "before it drops": I compare my thoughts to that of my never-ending playlist that would ensure I am listening to the tracks of my choosing. The more we press "repeat" button on a thought, the more it expands into similar thoughts and then klunk-klunk-klunk, it keeps dropping in our subconscious mind, forming a belief we carry around a particular issue in our lives. It is not a probability, but a certainty that you will be impacted by what you allow your subconscious to carry. It is so unbiased that you are served whatever you seek. It is so unbiased that everything is legal. It is so unbiased that you can imagine exist... So *"before it drops"* means that even though I may allow a Thought to go through my mind, I don't have to give it a comfortable seat to lounge and play video games with me and start a conversation. No way! When you notice an unpleasant Thought coming, knocking, be aware that your subconscious mind has been trained to open the doors and invite them, but you are also a free Being, with freewill to shut the door, with the understanding that no one will judge you. You cannot possess Christ Consciousness without feeling FREE.

How can unpleasant thoughts burden a free person? It is not possible... not a Christ Conscious mind. The Christ we know in the bible was never burdened by problems, no matter how horrible an affliction appeared in the human mind. When confronted with sickness, He offered healing; not from outside, but from within. He was an embodiment of healing. When you embody a concept, you become that concept. You are what you believe; so it doesn't come from another Source that you need to get permission from, no, you give yourself permission to express it... from within you. As a result it has the potential to be in continuous flow... if you are not-so distracted by outside predicament.

Isn't that neat???

Isn't it wonderful how we are created – to be an embodiment of solutions? It means everything we face in terms of problems, dangers, predicaments, afflictions, suffering, anguish, or any hardships here on earth have the potential to be resolved with Christ Consciousness. So next time you are enamored by Thoughts banging on the door of your consciousness, remember that you have this body but your Spirit is HIGH and LIFTED UP. Next time you are bombarded by the illusion of problems or general issues of life, do not make your eyes the main instrument to determine your reality. You are more than what your eyes can see. Therefore, redirect your awareness, raise your focus, go beyond, and know that you are guided and loved.

Say this with me:

Things are always working out for me.

I am co-creating a magical life.

I am living a life of abundance.

I am successful and happy.

I don't have to rely on my eyes all the time.

Things are not always what they seem

Things are ALWAYS working out for my good...

I have noticed time and time again that redirecting my focus helps me "uproot" some of those thoughts that are like weeds – those that would have otherwise embedded deeper in my subconscious – that part of my mindset that has become so used to accepting the "old-story" as norm without questioning...

Our subconscious mind will keep all kinds of data we have been gathering about our self-image, food, activities etc. Have you ever wondered why you think of eating a particular delicious meal and your mouth just salivates? I bet you're salivating right now as I mention ripe succulent peach. I'm just mentioning peach instead of pizza because I don't want to torture you, but think for a moment as you s-l-o-w-l-y bite into a big ripe peach, the juice dripping all over your fingers... you lick it and love the taste so much you take a bigger bite, lick it again and again because you cannot bear to let go of any ounce of that sweet juice. . . You know why you are salivating right now? Because your subconscious once recorded what it feels like

124

to eat sweet ripe peaches; in my case, fresh from the farm.

There are times when you simply think about an object and you start seeing it everywhere. Let's do a simple exercise: wherever you are sitting right now, tell your Subconscious what color you would like to see. Within seconds, the color you choose in your mind will start popping up everywhere around you.

Do you see it?

You see another one?

And another one?

I am sitting in the car right now parked under a tree, typing on my laptop. My daughter is taking a nap in the backseat and the weather is absolutely gorgeous. There are not that many red objects around here but guess what? My subconscious mind immediately directed my eyes towards the dashboard to see (1) the mileage pin, (2) the red part of a seat belt where you click, (3) my daughter's quilt, which is multi-color but has red flowers in it. You get the point, don't you? I chose the color red and here it came popping even in a place I hardly thought I would find it. Anything you seek your subconscious is sooooo freakishly redunkilosly (that's a made-up word) smart to find and bring it to you, for you to experience.

Oh dear subconscious, what a WONDER YOU are!!!

At this moment, I have been immediately transported back to childhood memories in my home-country school in Cameroon where we always sang. Now when I sing the song the song I just remembered, I no longer envision the blonde-hair, blue-eyed physical Jesus figure. Now I know better. I know my power – that "JESUS" really represents my Spirit or Divine Mind; so I *swap the word "Jesus" with a re-directed focus to my Divinity.*

You are free to sing along if you know the song, but if you're not familiar with it, simply give the words the meaning you prefer so that it rings true for you – that's the point of singing songs – that the words stir meaningful, supportive, intuitive, genuine and deep responses!

S-w-e-e-t, sweet Jesus (My Divine Mind)

Sweet Jesus (My Divine Mind)

What a wonder you are.

You are brighter than the morning star,

You are fairer, yes fairer,

Than the lily that grows by the wayside

You are precious, more precious than Gold. . .

Sorry about that digression, but my heart felt like singing and my Divine Mind knows what a Wonder I AM!!!!!!!!!!!!!

Alright, where were we??

Ok, subconscious: Oh the wonders you can do, because of the Wonder of Your Mind…

~Chapter Ten~

SEEK & FIND

Flowing with less resistance

"…and I said to my body, softly: 'I want to be your friend.' It took a long breath and replied: 'I have been waiting my whole life for this.'" ~Anonymous

I guess all this singing about Christ consciousness fits right into the next topic: "Seeking". I would liken this to finding the track (like a train) to align with your highest good so that when you're off, your Energy will announce for you to adjust. Like water going with the flow, you can live a life of intention by offering as little resistance as possible… and that's Not impossible.

Are you familiar with those words: *"seek and ye shall find"*? It is so simple and straight-forward that it can very easily be missed. Yet it can be a HUGE turning point for someone who gets IT. I think Jesus (Higher Consciousness) says it with absolute clarity -- When you seek it, you will find it: What you think you are seeking is also seeking you like a magnet; and you will *find* the essence of it in your experiences by hook or by crook. It is an established Universal Law: The things that you keep bringing up in your conversations and emotions, influenced by your beliefs, will summon similar forces to match your vibration and show up in your life. In other words, when you seek it, the Spirit realm will comply with you at a deep level and answer your *request*. This includes your speechless declarations or commands. Keep in mind that The Universe doesn't need words to communicate. God doesn't speak English or Italian. God is spirit and speaks in spirit anyway -- that silent still small voice FROM your soul.

People have been trained in religious circles to

bang their heads in prayers, crying out begging for blessings, and most of them don't know that they are actually seeking more desperation. You don't need loud desperate theater to get God's attention. In fact to get the attention of the Most High or gain clarity from a Higher /Divine perspective, God wants you to be STILL. In stillness, there is harmony as you seek and FEEL the Energy of your desires without distraction. In stillness, it is easier to listen and get to the point where it feels so true that you cannot be convinced otherwise. In other words what you see in spirit while you are still, you stand a high chance to accept it into your mind and express it.

Fear on the other hand comes with a squad of noisy chatty 'friends' such as feelings of inadequacy, worry, doubt, insecurity, to distract you from your track.

Spirit GPS:

Spirit GPS is the Divine presence (or signaling device) within you that conjures the path of least resistance. In many instances of healing, in scriptures, I noticed that Christ chose to go with less drama or little effort to do amazing things in people's lives. What that tells me is that suffering is not necessary when we are told in spirit what to do outside. But what happens with people when the Spirit (Christ Consciousness) reveals the path with the least amount of struggle? Our logical minds immediately jump in to dispel or audit it to prove that it cannot be that easy, joyful, pleasurable, exciting... And when people submit to the logical mind, they seek complicated ways to solve something that Spirit suggested could have been done with fewer struggles.

Excitement and joy rank high in the spirit preferred signaling device (Spirit GPS). Happy inspired Thoughts tell you where to put your attention next -- to follow your bliss: meaning you want happiness, peace, abundance, expansion, freedom out of the experiences you seek. The question I have been asking these days is that "if everything is already at our disposal in the Spirit realm, why do we have to fight so hard to get it?

Could it be part of our upbringing or slave generation conditioning?

Could it be part of the 'Old Testament' mentality that reveres fighting battles to gain victory?

Could this be a militant religious mindset we as a society are trained to accept?

I don't see Jesus (Christ Consciousness) ever fighting with swords and spears. If at all you find it in scriptures, please let me know. I rather saw Jesus accomplishing miracles with the power of the mind. He escaped many times from the crowd to BE STILL, MEDIATE and put Faith into action to bring changes. Could it be He knows the secret that the subconscious mind is always at our service when you seek, BE STILL and KNOW?

See LIFE ~ Seek ideals:

There is life in every idea...

So, the question I often ask when I encounter precious revelation is that: what am I going to do with this powerful knowledge?

Good question right? Have you ever asked that kind of question when you seek and find knowledge or a tool that seem to offer the right solutions? What are we supposed to do with what obviously makes changes imminent?

Well, if we're going to be creating anyway, I say there is no better time than now to seek new and improved lifestyle, not dead things of old. Now is the time to seek IDEALS that offer the path of *least resistance*. The subconscious mind may need frequent training to see, feel and accept the NEW ideals in order to get used to getting MORE out of life; but it is doable. If you are open to some ideas I have implemented in my own life to SEE my ideals come to pass, I don't mind sharing... that is what we are here for right?

Hey, it doesn't hurt to do simple things like

these examples i.e. if any resonates with you:

- Put a picture of a slimmer you in a frame next to your bed, where you see it every time – when yuo wake up and when you go to sleep. It will become part of your subconscious mind and your rational mind will find ways to bring that subconscious image into reality by altering your priorities and behaviors. Talk positive about yourself to yourself.

- Talk about the awareness of your good health, your radiant body instead of the diseases in your family. What you hear yourself say about you will come upon you.

- The reason you get no result is that you do not put the right emotions from your soul into it. Your whole being has to feel what you seek, so being lukewarm or nonchalant is only disconnecting you from that spirit. *Remember that your Soul understands the language of emotions.*

- Sit in a quiet place, put out your intention or thoughts regarding what is significant in your life right now; then ask your Inner-Being/ God/ Spirit within to align your thoughts with the emotions that affect results. You are the master of your Soul and your subconscious mind will yield to that message. Act on your impulsive force that feels blissful.

- Be alert: *What are you saying to you about YOU?*
Every day, my health is improving.

Every day my waistline is shaping?

Every day my features are forming nicely.

Every day life is getting better for me.

Do you BELIEVE what you are saying to you about you? All that is required of you to program your mind is to belief and feel the emotion that your "belief" ignites.

Fresh new job:

We are expansive, that's our nature! We cannot be stagnant and be happy about it; No way! I have not yet met that person who was in the same position as they were a year or two ago and was so satisfied that they were not seeking some form of improvement. I believe your health, your waistline, your bank account and your life will get a boost if you don't resist the idea of giving your mind a fresh new job to do. Our minds love it when we stretch it. Our minds love when we play those 'games' of expansion. I call it the "what if" or "Imagine if" game.

If I were The Mind right now I would be saying *"oh what is better than for me to imagine stuff and get happy?"*

I encourage you to play this game and imagine wild things as a way of stretching your mind beyond the norm. Think of something bigger than you have always thought before. Make it so big it scares the bonkers out of you or excites the lights out of you. Ooohh la la, I can imagine your subconscious mind jumping for joy... And if you just let your body PLAY along with that energy, you are sure to experience a shift in your mood, which is always beneficial in ways we may not recognize at this hot-minute. I consider my mind a playful friend and when I do the "imagine if" game with her, she gets so keyed-up and energized that I can't help but FEEL energetic as well. When you get into this wonderland of dreams with your subconscious mind, don't hold back the urges to see yourself in high places regarding of what you wish to manifest. The mind is a force that is part of our Being swirling fast and high to rock our world. But you can catch the bliss when you slow it down and FEEL that it could be true for you too. There is no need imagining things so hasty that you don't feel it as a possibility in your own life. You have at your disposal such powerful energies that seek every day to be activated and animated. When you start FEELING the energy with intensity, then you will realize that you have been sitting on HOLY ground all along. You will notice the magic IN you and the resources around you; which are Oh so ready to work with you and take you places to reach your potential.

Get ready... Get your mind ready and your body will be ready... No brainer!

WARNING: You are manifesting.

You are your own manifestation.

Seek... enjoy what you find!!!

~Chapter Eleven~

JOY-Personified

Fly Your Hedonist Flag

Warnings and side effects:

Laughter Is Totally Utterly Free Medicine!

Consume (unlimited) dose with gladness!

The more you laugh, the crazier you look, but crazy is the new

GENIUS hahaoooaoaiiiiohahahaaaaa ...

Consume at your own risk of enJOYment.

Laughter may cause you to relax more & have fun.

You may lose your ability to take life too seriously.

Too much happiness!!!

Joy is your 'Mojo'

Peace is your magic!

Joy is so important in our lives that one of the fruits of the spirit is dedicated to JOY. When your spirit is not entangled in worries, joy is always willing to dominate. But is it up to you – it starts with you and ends with you. Empowering, isn't it? Joy is not fleeting happiness influenced by a particular situation, rather it is gladness of the heart that is completely independent of the good or bad things that happen.

JOY IS HEALING energy and it is no surprised that it is referred to as "GOOD MEDICINE" *(proverbs17:22)*. Repressed emotions *dry up the bones* or cause physical blockages in the body. When joy energy is not allowed to flow, not allowed to be expressed through your body temple, your bones and joints feel the tension usually exhibited as pain, such as arthritis. It is very important for your mind and body to be allowed access to the spirit of Joy. I say 'ACCESS' because no one is without it – joy dwells as energy within every soul. It just needs to be embodied and fully expressed.

JOY IS STRENGTH that allows us to fix our gaze on the inner supernatural fortitude rather than on the circumstances. All it requires of you is for your mind to accept it and you will show up during hard times with smiles and confidence, ruling your life from that Sacred space of supernatural gladness. It is well documented that several brain centers—especially the pleasure center moves us to remember pleasurable experiences not just for the sake of pleasure, but for the healing and strengthening it brings. The brain produces endorphins, which are opium-like compounds the brain secretes to heighten pleasure that lifts us above pain and emotional suffering... and these brain centers can be triggered into activity by practicing meditation, laughter, mindful breathing, dancing or stretching. If I had no other reason but to alleviate pain at will, I say the JOY deserves a major dwelling place in my life.

Since the feeling world inside you was designed to have an effect on your behavior and body, your body naturally has a mechanism in place to respond to your sense of wellbeing. It is simply magical to witness what joy can accomplish. When you ALLOW your cells to live in this space of Joy and Peace; you radiate a happy version of you more effortlessly, more rapidly, more often. Every thought you think has unique emotions attached to it, so if you wish to change your feelings of frustration to that of exuberant passion, then you have to change what you are thinking and voila! The same issues that used to irritate you or things that used to make you feel like a failure will turn into ingenious adventures. Don't be surprised when the happy, positive thoughts activate energies that make you smile to yourself, sing to yourself, put springs on your steps and make you rejoice like you can conquer the world. That is the Spirit of JOY in action – actually conquering emotional states of depression, frustration, anxiety etc. This stuff is fo'real yo! (speaking in my playful voice). But seriously, this is not just a Law of Attraction gibberish that is made up to sound good. It actually has remarkable mental and emotional effects that if mastered, will make a world of difference in your health. Thoughts alone can stir you up to do things that were once limiting your progress. The more you give yourself the priceless gift of feeling the high energy of joy, the more your cells will thank you reveal your inner glow.

You cannot be joyful and bored at the same time. Almost impossible!!!!!!! There is tremendous energy build-up in a person who exudes joy – they not only laugh more, but CREATE more. Yes, I strongly believe that laughter itself is a creative spirit: Not only does it heal but pumps you with more energy that allows you to partake in the beauty of molding an ordeal into amazing adventure. Now that's GENUIS!!!

Ready to be bombarded with inspiration and build momentum?

The Spirit called JOY, which ranks at the top of the "emotional guidance scale" as having strong attraction-factor, is in alignment with your innate freedom. You are born with it. Joy is known for delivering inspiration to your being. Since this spirit doesn't come from anywhere else but within, the good news is that everyone is absolutely capable of finding inspiration to do, be and have more out of life. When your attitude is set on entertaining positive happy thoughts, similar thoughts will be attracted to those initial happy thoughts that will build momentum feeding on other happy thoughts, opening up channels in your Soul that make you feel like you belong to another dimension. Yes, when you're not fixated on controlling cerebral aspects of life, you're neither burdened nor restrained. Now that is the level of freedom to revel in because therein lies your 'Angel' wings to FLY. FLY. FLY!

Sometimes you just need a freaking good laugh... to burn calories too! I'm not kidding you when I say laughter always makes me pee and the reason I am happy about that is because you know what that means – you are flushing out toxins. Okay fine, that may have been TMI (too much information) but the idea that laughter benefits health has been around for ages. Once again I totally agree with the scripture verse: *"a joyful heart is good medicine but a broken Spirit dries up the bone." (Proverbs17:22).* But ouch! Who wants desiccated bones?

Not me!

And I bet you wouldn't want that either.

So if it means you ought to go on a hunt every day and find reasons all around you to laugh, why not? There are enough things going on to make us clinch in the emotional bondage of sadness and anxiety. Go get yourself free doses of laughter and if you need more triggers, there are countless funny YouTube videos of silly things people do, you can watch a comedy show, revisit a very funny chapter of your life in your mind, call a sibling or friend who knows how to crack you up, even if you run the risk of wetting your pants. There she goes again with the "pee joke"... But it's TURE :-))

All I'm saying is, be intentional about attracting humor at will, to constantly raise your vibration. There can be an element of fun in pretty much anything you observe. You just have to look beyond what everyone normally calls it; and that requires an open mind. Laughter has been researched, studied and documented in many scientific publications demonstrating the immediate and assessable usefulness in life:

- *It stretches our facial muscles*

- *Boosts our heart rate*

- *Reduces stress*

- *Reduces muscle tension*

- *Raises energy expenditure*

- *Promotes relaxation and good sleep*

- *Prompts our bodies to produce more T-cells, thus boosting the immune system*

- *Produce happy chemicals (endorphins) in the brain*

- *The harder we laugh, the faster we breathe thereby sending more oxygen to our tissues. And get this: Our brain will respond to laughter even if the laughter is faked.*

Wow! The list of benefits ain't no joke!

Who knew it was so healthy to laugh your lungs out!!! It gives me so many reasons to think about ways to start, spend and end my day with laughter as a companion. I also invite you to feel free "giggling-your-brains" (whatever that means LOL) and snort if you have to. Really, if this news doesn't trigger the need for you to start grinning from ear to ear, I may be tempted to come over and start a tickle-fight with you.

Oh wait, there's more... Some studies even indicated the amount of calories you could actually burn laughing: Ten (10) minutes of hearty laughter not only affords you the aforementioned health benefits, but could burn approximately fifty calories. Hey, 50 calories may sound minimal but if I nibble a piece of chocolate, or squeeze extra mayonnaise into my sandwich, not to mention the plantain chips I just ate, it counts for something.

There are people who actually practice Laughter Therapy. Can you tell I am already loving this "THERRA'py" idea?

Yes, I inserted my name in there because I'm a BEliever. It's funny that I am writing this chapter on laughter on the day I watched some hilarious YouTube clips my sister shared about African parenting. Oh I laughed so hard you can guess what happened... haha! I don't know how it all transpired into me writing on this topic because it wasn't my plan to write the JOY chapter today. I was actually looking forward to organizing some notes I jotted about another subject but when I put my daughter down for a nap, turned on my computer, I felt drawn to the theme of JOY and LAUGHTER. I had no notes planned but as I started typing, ideas came flowing. Not long after that my daughter woke up from her short nap and I took her out to the mall to play in the indoor playground. It was FUN watching her enjoying herself and especially those her little friends in the 'still-learning-to-run' stage. We returned home and my sister texted me a video clip to watch. My goodness, did I have a good laugh or what?

I am very sure I attracted those hilarious clips into my experience. My son was in the basement playing when he heard my laughter. He came running up the stairs to find out why Mama was having a laughing-fit. By the time he made it to the family room, the clip had ended. He begged me to replay so that he too could experience the amusement. I tell you laughter is INFECTIOUS!!! I replayed it for his pleasure (and mine of course);

and he laaaaaughed at everything that was being said. But you have to understand that he is a second-grader, born and raised in America and he doesn't quite understand any of the jokes on African parenting style; but because I was hysterically helplessly shedding tears of pure joy, he couldn't resist the energy.

Laugh more, toil less. It's the way to insane freeeeeedom

Don't be afraid of your own light. Laughter is light. It lights up the cells in your body. It is actually hard on you physically to be dragging around emotional baggage throughout the day, not to talk of weeks, months and years; but people typically don't make that connection. However when you get it, you will want to slap yourself for ever feeling bad about trivial things. Women, Moms especially should not hesitate to cut some slacks because you don't need to put yourself under unnecessary stress. Who needs stress when life is waiting for you to live?

*Life is waiting for you to roll on the floor and *laugh your wonderful self to bliss.

*Life is waiting for you to float in ecstasy.

*Life is waiting for you to dance your muscles to painful breakthroughs and flexibility.

*Your inner-lover is waiting to bask in a wild and tender fantastically-enchanting and serene scene in the middle of nowhere.

*Life is waiting for you to charge your electric force and freely dance your intoxicating beauty until you can hear the Angels chanting!

Life is not about work-work and barely play; no way! Your soul already knows the truth that work-work-work only grants you a dull, uninteresting stressful life. Ladies, don't feel guilty for cancelling some obligations. Take some things off your plate and free up time for fun activities that boost your mood...that is, if your 'job' doesn't already give you that. This is one of the major inspirations behind the creation of my African fitness/wellness coaching program called SAKKACISE. Like most mothers, I cherish the idea of giving. I love giving my time and energy to others but I would rather be giving from OVERFLOW. This has a lot to do with learning to be selfish (or what I call Sacred Selfishness) which means I make sure to fill up my own cup first; because I don't want to be that person who is always exhausted and providing from deficient energy. Moms, who are ever so busy giving to others need to be more intentional about their souls' needs first and foremost. So the golden question is: How?!?

For me, it begins with a simple question I ask myself daily: **What does my soul need today?**

Sometimes, it just means finding an outlet to

release my stress: soak in some Epsom salt lavender infused bathtub for as longgggg as I can afford to, find ways to uplift my spirit, feed my soul: connect with nature, read a book, listen to music, engage in "mental-sex" with my Awakened friends, push myself beyond 'poor-me' lazy moods and conduct fun activities, such as SAKKACISE and of course, meditate. It takes as much time and energy to boost my mood as it does to sulk in "poor-me'ness".

Who is poor? Not this Goddess!!! Every soul is already free to choose joy, light, peace, abundance of energy... It is just matter of tapping into that ocean of delight.

She called me hedonist:

One day I received a text from my friend who said something to the effect of *"Finally"!!! I finally figured you out; you are a Hedonist.*

I read her text and for a minute I got confused because I thought the word hedonist was an insult. Hahahahahaahahaahaaa... Ohh, the things that happen when you have intellectual friends rocking your world and painting your days with laughter-infused-confusion. This proves that perception is the ruler of your mood and attitude towards life.

I absolutely love the google definition of hedonist: *a person who believes that the pursuit of pleasure is the most important thing in life...*

One thing to note is that seeking pleasure in life is clearly a choice. People who make that choice face the same difficulties that everyone on the planet faces. Of course your battles might be different from mine but as long as you live this life, sooner or later you will discover that no one lives without some form of adversity. Many people that have crossed my path in life have assumed that I lead a perfect life, until I open up and enlist some of the challenges I have faced since childhood, to teenage years, adulthood and motherhood... then they realize "oh, your 'happy-go-lucky' attitude is really a choice.

I remember a group chat we had with a friend who was not willing to let go of a painful experience and she posed the question: "How do you forgive? I cannot ask good for those who hurt me. I don't like this *forgiveness-thing'.* Is there any other way?"

What I told her is what I have practiced in my life. I believe that we all (even pleasure-seekers) have been hurt and lied to and manipulated; but I don't think anchoring ourselves down with the spirit of resentment is the way forward. I sincerely responded the only way I know I live my life:

"*When you choose not to forgive, you are on the opposite side of freedom i.e. you are blocking your own Joy, sabotaging your right to freely live a happy life. If you don't want to interact with those who hurt you, it is your right; but YOU are the creator of your realities and holding on to the pain is a form of interacting with them and continuing to hurt yourself. No one ever felt*

FREE and experienced JOY by harboring bitterness. Letting go of the pain YOU feel is not a sign of weakness; rather it takes self-love and resolve. Forgiving others is a sure way to FREE yourself from that bondage of hatred. It takes go(o)d attributes IN you – (i.e. your God-Self in action) and by doing what is GOOD, you are honoring the GOD in you. You are allowing LOVE to rule and dominate your decisions; and love never fails. On the other hand, the unforgiving spirit only invites resentment; one of the energies that will surely halt your creative flow and manifestations. All in all, forgiving your enemies is for your own sake – to be FREE... to manifest GO(O)D and HAPPY days ahead!!!

Need I say more?

What is better than being FREE to manifest MORE GOODness in your life?

Oh, I want that for you so much that I even composed a simple, easy to remember poem. You can print and paste it in a place where you can see and read every day sunrise displays its bright rays; as a gentle reminder of your innate spirit of JOY:

Don't get mad, think glad

Don't get bored, Choose Joy

Don't get cranky, BE happy

Laugh your lungs out. Oh, ever so loud

Laugh all you can

It's FREE medicine

And it's all within!

~Chapter Twelve~

The Energy of YES

The creative power of your Goddess kingdom within always says "Yes" to what your soul needs - "Yes" to you discovering the path of least resistance. "Yes" to taking you to the portal that leads you to your dreams. It is a very liberating feeling. But beware... beware of fear... As you know, success in anything you wish to achieve is a journey of discovery; but Fear will keep reminding you about failure, time, impossibilities, scarcity and even despair. Don't be surprised if along the way you hear such thoughts popping like corn:

"what if something bad happens"?

"What if I'm not able"

"What if I fall along the way"

And the big one: "What will people say?"

Whenever your thoughts say things like "I am not good enough yet" or "I may fail", know that you have the power to generate thoughts that are beyond that stinking level of thinking. The universal laws don't demand perfection; rather it is about evolution – shifting your awareness to discover layers and heights of your own health, wellness, freedom and yes, greatness.

The Energy of YES feels liberating!

Can you think of anyone who would say No to total wellbeing? But when you discount the "YES Energy" you are essentially saying you don't want an improved life. As you move with the energy of your 'YES' you will be surprised at the doors that will fling open for you. Your intention to move forward day by day has enough Force to make pathways where there were once walls. Since the law of attraction is pure non-discriminative energy flowing where it is being magnetized, what you're emotionally capable of conjuring is what you magnify. So when you respond to your own calling with a resounding profound "YES-mood", the light of your greatness will begin to shine brighter than your excuses, and the more you'll pulsate with the rhythm of your desires. You'll attract people of similar energies. They will be drawn to the vicinity of your energy regardless of your race, gender or background; and whenever high energies come together and mingle, the probability of boosting and pumping your actions goes Up many degrees higher... thus amazing results.

Does it take practice?

Absolutely! But the practice is the fun process: the ecstasy of discovering what a thrilling life you can live. FUN is a choice, you know... so is executing your Power of YES!!!

The other "F" Word: FOOD & Wellness Awareness

Food. Food. Food. Oh the almighty food. If you ask the question "what is in food?', the answer you get will often depend on who you ask and where you perform your search. But we can all agree that food is an edible, digestible substance which consists of nutritious elements that are essential for life. These nutrients have healing properties that generate energy and foster our body's vitality, radiance and growth. However, food isn't all of that anymore because we live in the age where it has been corrupted to have addictive and destructive components...

That said, food was never meant to have power over you. It doesn't have to consume you; you consume it!! Food can only play the healing role in full capacity after *you have established confidence in your own power!*

Your inner strength and conviction of what you want out of your relationship with food is what maps out the transformation journey. In the process of releasing old beliefs, you also release your old attachment to food that can corrupt the New version of you. When your focus has shifted from old beliefs and habits to what you have to gain instead, your consciousness and your mouth work together; and the manner in which you approach food after this stage is very different - keyword 'different'. You will realize your whole experience of eating is no longer polluted with judgment-calls that make you feel bad. Even your negative thoughts will become opportunities for you to attempt critical thinking – the type of thoughts that catapult you into seeking solutions rather than blaming and shaming your self-image.

In this new state of awareness regarding wellness, you eat and savor your well-chosen meals with respect and appreciation – it could be respect for your body-temple, your cells, or just immense appreciation for where you are in your journey, or the wonderful person that You KNOW you are made to BE!

~Chapter Thirteen~

Appreciation

Affects How

You Care

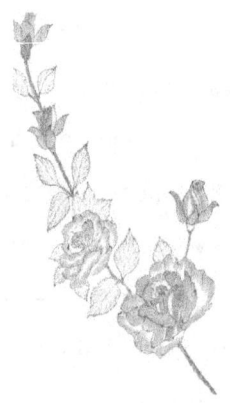

When your heart is grateful for something or

someone, you admire and take care of them. ~Therra

Buddha puts it this way: *"If we could see the miracle of a single flower clearly, our whole life would change."*

I came across Buddha's profound words when I was already an adult, but a quick flash back takes me to when I was a teenager stretching this rose flower, I was very intrigued beyond the surface attributes of the flower. It's been more than two decades but I still recall the feeling, examining the flower thinking *"how did the formation of these petals align so perfectly, yet seem like they're going in different directions?"* If you observe roses in full bloom or just a single stem closely, you will realize it has irresistible silky soft petals and the fragrance is so alluring you won't resist touching it or get into closer proximity to sniff its aroma. The stem on the other hand has sharp thorns that aren't as gentle to the touch – the stem is very thorny and rough. However what we commonly recall and say about a rose flower is not a single part, but the entire plant as a masterpiece that makes a beautiful statement, be it in a vase or in the garden.

That flower is not different from YOU. It is part of your existence, telling the story of YOU; that **You Are Also A Masterpiece,** created by the same Almighty Universal Mind.

Accept your Wholeness!

Self-Love is the acceptance of my uniqueness, weirdness,
foolishness and wholeness!

Accept your wholeness AND then build a relationship that appreciates your wholeness, for you are perfect! Whatever you fully accept, you also allow yourself to see beyond its surface. By making the decision to accept something, you are opening your mind up to know about it. This is how knowing 'Of' something at first can lead to forming a long lasting relationship. When you have a good impression of yourself and you establish a good relationship, discovering more about you becomes a thrill. The more eagerness you bring into your self-discovery the more you break your own barriers and free yourself to see the different aspects of your Being. It is absolutely wonderful to be interested in knowing more about you because seeing the magnificence of your whole Being grants you knowledge of how high and far you can go. As you sharpen your relationship between your physical and Spirit-Self, you learn quickly to take advantage of your balance, brilliance, creativity and unstoppable nature. It is this deep connection with your True identity that gives birth to courage. Courage in itself is an offering of sincere gratitude, deep rooted in the truth that there is more beyond your flesh. And the more you pour your own words of courageous self-appreciation into your life, the more you find ways to treat yourself with care.

Like a rose flower,
It takes courage to soften your heart,
accept your thorns and live your truth,
but it solidifies your relationship with your soul
and the people who appreciate your wholeness!

I love BE-ing grateful

I love being grateful.

And I think gratitude loves me too.

It puts me in an elevated state that explodes my frustrations into poetic mosaic and gets me smiling in the

present tense!

The practice of gratitude is a quality that brings us in harmony with the *present* moment. In the present moment a grateful heart is not concerned about right or wrong doings, what I have done or didn't do, but simply appreciating all, just the way it is. It means as I rise every day, nothing can stop me from starting over and living the life of my choosing. This awareness stops pressing the replay button on past guilt or mistakes because it is focused on my value and worth as a person, which in a way is telling the Universe:

- *I AM happy with who I AM and no matter where I am, the state of my spirit is what matters. I AM at ease with myself, but I AM also ready for more...*

Because the past is over. NOW is the time to

start recording your future with superb bliss in mind. Doesn't that sound more fun? From here it can only be more of what you wish because your intention is set to find less to criticize or devalue about you, and more to appreciate.

NOW is......
Any*time*, Any*where*

If Now is the time to BE happy, then the Creator that you are is the one who is responsible for creating that reality. The practice of gratitude is a simple technique that you can do anywhere and at any time. No longer should TIME be a reason why you cannot do something that may calm your nerves, boost your mood, make you happy and affect real transformation in your life. Your wellbeing depends on happiness, so it should be worth your time here on earth to pursue a lively, dynamic, winning lifestyle starting with the present/Now: whenever, whenever, whenever...

Did you know (of course you know) that

happiness also plays a HUGE, HUMONGOUS, GIGANTIC-TITANIC role in your body and cells? Happiness is not just about emotional balance but it affects how your cells behave in your system; and you know what can prove it? Your energy level!!! How our cells react positively to a HAPPY MOOD is something that is well documented and established even in medical circles; and studies have shown that Gratitude has a lot to do with it. So then, why do we, especially women, choose to suppress happiness due to Self-criticisms? Why does it have to be so hard to intentionally direct your life towards the Ease that Happiness brings? The Truth is that every single one of us deserve to be happy. We all deserve to create a healthy life but that cannot be manufactured in a factory. Happy and healthy can only be activated from within; that is just the way it is, and has ALWAYS been. A seed is never seen under the soil but it bears fruits. Likewise the secret to happiness is to focus your thoughts on things that make you feel good in your spirit. Lack of happiness is dryness and nothing grows in a dry place; if at all anything grows, it is sparse and characterized by scarcity!

Make your life an expression and declaration of the abundance that happy and healthy brings. If that is what you believe in, it will show. I have noticed in my own experience that expressing my appreciation brings the feeling of relaxation that paves the way for a shift in vibration and heightens my admiration for my beauty, health, weight or whatever else I am prone to take for granted. In the flow of such energy, I am pumped and inspired to take action; promoting my wellbeing. It is through appreciation that you can easily practice to revamp your sense of worthiness. When you are feeling worthy, you quickly notice that fighting with what you hate is waste of time, for it will only keep attracting energy that gets you stuck. But a wise Goddess knows better – she doesn't struggle when she can switch to appreciation-mode and proudly celebrate her worth. Knowing this and living this as your Truth frees you to live apart from what anyone thinks of you. The only opinion that counts is Yours.

A great bonus called:
CLARITY.

The Art of paying attention and taking notice of how the Universe is responding to you is a love affair. The keyword here is NOTICE because the Universe has been responding all along but while you were caught up in looking at and analyzing your struggles, you couldn't SEE what was in you the whole time. You could not notice all these things you're now grateful for and could hardly bring yourself to acknowledge the Goddess that you are. But now that your soul is vibrating with the frequency of love and appreciation, you are attracting more to be grateful for. This forms a very sweet reciprocal relationship with your essence that brings answers to your needs.

In this simple exercise you can do anywhere and at any time to keep attracting what you want, even your cells will have something happy to say –

I can bet my fresh carrot juice on that.

DO this exercise, say it aloud:

"I appreciate YOU for

ALWAYS being there for me."

Now stop and think: Who are you appreciating?

You are appreciating the Divine Source, your co-creative partner, the Goddess in you, your Soul, your True Self.

Create time to be alone for about 10-15 minutes a day or whatever suits you. The location doesn't matter; it could be during your break at work, on your ride home (if you take public transportation or have a chauffeur), in a restaurant, at the airport/ airplane, in your home . . . you get the point.

If yes, get a pen, an iphone or any writing device and WRITE down what you LIKE and APPRECIATE about YOU. It could be just looking at yourself in the mirror, that is, if you like mirrors like I do. If you choose a mirror as part of your exercise, stand facing yourself in full length. When you notice anything such as excess weight, giggly parts, rolls and flabby-flabbazzo on display on your skin, say "that's okay; it is just an indicator of a vibration that needs to change." And be thankful for that awareness.

I remember doing this mirror exercise during my postpartum days (I still do it) and noticing all my stretch marks and extended tummy and rubbing it I said *"hello there, wow, so here we are... No worries, we are going make it and we're gonna rock this body and shine together."*

You see, you can totally control your focus, your perception and countenance. You can appreciating whatever you are faced with. It is harder on your cells to condemn and frown than to smile, you know that right? Beating yourself up, criticizing, complaining, judging, blaming is like banging your head on a concrete wall and expecting no pain. Sorry but guilt-trips only produce counter-productive results, so be easy on yourself. You will find that the JOY-full vibration keeps you stimulated and motivated to be an indestructible creative force (that you really are).

Every time you notice and acknowledge something coming from the Source of love and abundance, it's almost as if Angels increases the frequency, probability and rapidity of bringing that thing into your life. And a time will come when you'll suddenly realize Oh my freaking God, my skinny jeans fit!!! You know why? It is because the vibration of love and abundance is not caught up in the struggle of fighting against anything; so you are flowing with the waves of loving the process. As you allow your vibration increase in frequency, your awareness is expanding and you will just want to keep appreciating everything because your re-NEW-ed awareness sees value in everything.

What you appreciate, appreciates!

Gratitude is an amazing mood-changer and mind-altering exercise. I bought a board from the office supply store and brought it home and called

"GRATITUDE IS THE ATTITUDE" Board. It was aimed at getting my whole family into the FUN of writing and posting what makes their heart glad on any given day. This helps to direct our minds towards the things that will uplift our Spirit and boost our attitude about life. The tool makes focusing on manifesting lighthearted without being too conscious of the serious business of manifesting. Some people take it too seriously and lose the essence of what the process can do to our cells, mind, emotions and bodies. The whole purpose is JOY and without joy, you lose strength to keep up.

- Sit quietly for 5 minutes and ask God to send hosts of Angels to guide you, give you clues all day long. This attitude opens up your creative juices to know that there is another day, another chance. You may not know the method that God will bring your motivation, so be open and have fun with it!

APPRECIATION from

You to You:

My beloved body, I acknowledge you are my teacher and I'm so thankful that you are teaching me to discern what I truly want in obvious ways.

- *Thank you my (even overweight) body! You were there for me when I needed pounds to carry our baby (if you're a Mom). You helped me meet and even exceed the range of weight gain recommendations.*

- *You gave me cushion all around my bones and muscles while I was pregnant. Thank you!*

BUT NOW...

I'm ready to move on... (Call your name), it is time to move on. It is time to experience other things and the satisfaction that comes with it. It is time to experience what this situation has caused me to desire. It is time to experience my desired size (name the size).

It is time to live a healthy, vibrant life.

I feel ready. I am ready (SMILE).

I can feel the energy flowing, yes!

I know I am ready (SMILE if you feel like it).

Yes! I know I am ready this time.

It is MY time to take this journey of transformation & Self-mastery and just enJOY!!!

~Chapter Fourteen~

My Desires

What is the underlying spirit within your desires?

Our very existence and experiences have already put oodles and oodles of desires into our hearts. We don't have to search long to find our desires staring us in the face because every single day on this planet adds to the previous list of desires we had yesterday. Our desire for happiness and wellbeing never ends. Our desire for wealth never ceases. Our desire for fulfilling relationships grows as we grow. Our desire for better career and financial stability always rises. Our desire for better health is constant... But we are also adorned with unique gifts to support our growing desires. Why would humans be created to have desires without the ability to manifest them? We've all heard it said that *"if you dream it, you can achieve it."* If you want to put your inborn gifts to good use, all you need to do is:

- *focus on caring about how you feel*

- *cultivate serenity within yourself*

- *believe you are worthy of what you desire*

- *let those good vibes (or feelings) guide you, and you are sure to discover how amazing you are created to be.*

The more you focus on nurturing yourself, the more you will be peeling off layers of those New ideas about your beautiful Spirit. Your Spirit is already Amazing! Don't let your mind or society use your circumstances or other aspects of your life to justify any scarcity. Everyone has their share of bumps and bruises but if you can still bring yourself to believe in the amazing nature of your spirit and actually embody that belief, your life will prove it.

Look at the following words, first, feel its truth and with conviction, say it loud:

I Am Amazing!

I Am Wonderful.

I Am Worthy.

I Am Secure.

I Am Happy.

I Am Resourceful.

I Am Free. (remember, make it personal, feel it and boldly declare: I Am Free!!!!!!!

You are here to live, not exist. You are created to be creative. The liveliness within you sparks creativity. Creating your reality is a Goddess's birthright. Yes, a Creative Goddess I AM, if I may say so myself. If no one ever told you that, well, you just heard me. All it takes for you now is to say YES to your Amazingly, wonderful, worthy, secure, happy, resourceful, free Self; and watch how that Energy becomes part of You:

Subconsciously You. Unapologetically You.

The Law of Attraction's doesn't discriminate what group of humans on this planet deserve more blessings based on religion or place of birth. The law of attraction deals with the rawness and realness of the energy that you authentically and profoundly hold as truths in your soul. If you feel it real in your heart and believe it to be true in your soul, then you most certainly will emit a different kind of energy than someone who is faking or saying it without depth. You cannot fake your deeper Truth, especially as your deeper Self can speak... even without words.

The energy of Self-love and confidence always produce a lighthearted aura, than the energy of Self-pity. Regardless of religious affiliation, energy IS energy. Whether you carry around the thickest bible, recite long verses, sing the loudest praise songs, attend an all-night church services, the law of attraction is responding to the underlying spirit from within.

It is very limiting to think that the Almighty

Universal Mind (God) will lower the standards of the laws that run the entire Universe to match only what members of a certain religious group prefer. When you give credit to a particular religion, you are down-playing the power of the Omnipresent, Omnipotent, Omniscient Divine Source we call God.

You can be anywhere in the world and attract this everlasting Energy. It is timeless. It is eternal. It never ends.

Once your intention is made known in the spirit realm; it doesn't regress or die just because the answer hasn't made an instant appearance in your life. It is very alive in spirit, but when you keep doubting your Divine ability to manifest it, you will obviously feel the conflict within you, and it will bring a noticeable degree of distress. That distress is trying to communicate something – how you perceive your conviction in relation to your Divine connection.

Your desire is spirit and yes, spirit is invisible but certainly not absent. Invisible doesn't mean lack thereof. In fact, the invisible is a very active part of your days, nights, habits and growth. My kids hardly ever see the ingredients I put in the crepes I make or a cake when it is already fully baked. But if you cut a slice and taste, you can tell the major ingredients. If it is over-salted or over-sweetened, you cannot tell from just looking at it... until you taste it. So don't ever ignore the invisible. In fact, be very selective about the invisible ingredients in your life than what outsiders see.

If you think more happy, healthy, beautiful, pleasant ideas, believe me, your need to fret will drastically reduce. This is the part that confuses people who focus with their naked eyes, without being aware that the larger invisible part of you (your ingredients). Your Spirit is a big part of the role you play here on planet earth. What your Spirit perceives and believes, your physical life and body will 'taste' exactly like it. That is just the way the Universe works: your life is a reflection of your inner perception. Hence never underestimate the role of the invisible -- In fact the reverse should be your focus: Take the physical aspects of your life such as your shape, size, health, even relationships as code of what you can magnify in your spirit.

In this unseen world of spirit, your thoughts travel like 'missile-speed' (for lack of better words). It doesn't take long for you to think a thought. Think about that, and you'll realize there is no time hindrance in what you just thought. You just have to choose from the abundance upon abundance of ideas and focus on the fulfillment.

So..... Are you ready to catch up?

What is the underlying spirit within your desires?

That is a question only YOU can answer! For me, the part that makes manifestation within the context of the law of attraction appealing is that you are never alone. You may have been told that being alone is a boring thing but for me, my thoughts are my friends... Keep in mind I said "My friends" – They are Not me, so I don't have to engage with every single thought that crosses my mind, or let them define me.

Your sixth-sense or instincts are very telling... Are you aware of what they want to tell you?

Be aware that:

- We are called to be co-creators with The Universal Mind. Did you hear that? Co-creators with The Omniscient. How can you limit that?

- God wants YOU to be part of the process. This means there is Divine power in every operation.

- There is Divine power in every operation.

- There is Divine power in every operation.

  Are you paying attention?

  Are you paying attention?

  Are you paying attention?

  If so, are you doing things just through action without the voice and wisdom of your instincts?

  These are good questions to ponder on...

- Are you focusing your energy on the positive outcome?

- Is what you are doing born of Love?

- Are you focused on gathering heaps of energy sucking excuses?
- Are you willing to give yourself permission to explore some of the benefits that the positive outcome might bring? (Then write down the benefits)
- Are YOU treating your life with lack of enthusiasm on the subject of what you really desire... thinking that your underlying instincts don't matter?

Always remember your worthiness:

It builds into your soul and when it becomes natural to the point where you don't doubt it, embodies you and stimulates your enthusiasm. You don't need to make other people see or acknowledge your worth because it is not their dream or prime preoccupation. It is something you have to readily accept or take your sweet time to grow into, but when you spend your time and days thinking that your wings are limited in any area, you obviously are opening up pathways to experience lack; which a worthy person doesn't identify with. It is that Simple; not easy to accept, but honest-to-God truth: The essence of the energy you use to focus is always moving towards a Point of attraction...........And you can tell, can't you?

Unfortunately, most people go on to waste years and decades of their lives focusing on the outside before realizing that it never works that way and will never work. There are blocks on multiple levels of your consciousness preventing you from ever feeling your best and reaching your ideal. If there is one thing I wish for you to take away from all of this, it's this: No amount of medication or pill will ever ensure your Wellbeing...It is an inner-game!

You must stir your eagerness to become comfortable dealing with the fundamental issues hidden beneath the surface to restore your wellbeing.

Your health is not outside.

I'm glad you are diving deeper.....

So next time your thoughts say: "I can't", remember to dig deep and feel "I can"

Everything you harvest correlates with the quality of your soil:

It is a well-established natural pattern in the Plant-Kingdom that before the plant ever shows its bud above ground level, there is a lot that goes on underneath the surface, after the seed is planted -- fertile soil constitutes nutrients that provide better nourishment to the seeds, which eventually yields bountiful harvest beyond what the dryness of drought can compare to.

The lesson for us humans who are aware of how nature works is that we continue to nourish our soil(soul) with loved-based energy, having full assurance that the Universe is unraveling your splendor. The Law of attraction is your creative cohort that makes it easy for you to detect the direction of your focus. Energy focused on dryness feels dull while your focus on fertility feels plentiful:

- *It FEELS BETTER to breathe, than to struggle.*

- *It FEELS BETTER to relax, than to grumble*

- *It FEELS BETTER to believe, than to be worried sick.*

- *It FEELS BETTER to create, than to freeze in regret.*

- *SMILE and RELEASE any bondage-feelings; because you're born to be FREE and FEEL GO(O)D!!!*

Do you ever sit, just sit... no cell phones, no TV, no Ipad... just you, making time to listen to your body languages? Body language doesn't just apply to your non-verbal behavior in social settings. Your body is an excellent communicator of what your cells are experiencing. The stress you feel is a 'voice' speaking on behalf of your cells when they are gasping for relief.

On the cellular level, you are a Being of **freedom and joy**, meaning your cells feel more at ease, at home, in their natural state when given room to express that freedom. Such a space allows them to carry out their important functions without hindrance. If you don't feel ease, relief or at peace from the experiences you allow into your life, then you are essentially saying: *"I Want More Dis-Ease"*.

Now, would you in your right senses wake up every day and announce that you want more diseases? Well, you don't have to do so verbally because your cells have a way of telling...

Sickness is a sign of imbalance within.

Feeling lethargic is a sign of imbalance.

Feeling burdened is definite imbalance within. Imagine in your gorgeous home you have a gold fish tank and one day you walk in to find your fish stuck in a muddy, dark tank.

How would you feel (for the fish) seeing that they are struggling for survival in the mud? Your cells are born in an environment where the energy of joy easily radiates with no "muddy" hindrances. Your weight gain, be it physical or emotional, is just a loud cry from your cells. They are tired of you strangling them in worries, tired of you binding them in fear and sick of you hiding them in shame. The thing keeping you from flaunting a fit, healthier body has nothing to do with food, as much as you would like to believe that so you can blame calories. Rather, as a being of freedom, you cannot function on a higher level without letting go of these 'sick-and-tired' energies. The sick-and-tired energies will only take you as far as "sick-and-tired can go – to activities and habits that don't contribute to your evolution.

Read that again.......

Have you noticed that your desire for wellness doesn't go away no matter how hard you try to shove it under the rug or pretend it is not bothering you? You may even run to the sweetness and comfort of ice-cream and doughnuts in an attempt to fill the 'void', but the nudges in your soul won't budge nor bow down to sweet treats. Food has never been known to satisfy any void you may be feeling, so food will never influence real sustainable change. A burdened mind, coupled with a sick, tired and stressed body make an awful environment for cells to live in. Your cells will never thrive in gloominess, never! Your cells cannot freely breathe when at the same time, you are suppressing your own progress. How will you set them free??

Using hints, Going one step at a time... The Art of Ascending

If one desires a change, one must be that change before that change can take place. ~Gita Bellin

I will replace the word 'change' with "ASCEND" because I wish for you to also come to terms with the notion that once you know how to truly rise above the 'problem', then you are no longer gripped by the concerns of the problem. It doesn't mean you are in denial or ignoring the situation, but you are dealing with it from an ascended perspective. The wisdom gained from that standpoint is like extra dose of renewed strength for you to rise even higher. With this awareness that the dwelling place (of your consciousness) has shifted, change feels more like adventure, instead of a challenge.

The more you recognize that life's circumstances don't just happen, but that your experiences are unfolding with the permission of your awareness, you would want to put yourself in a position where you are focused and relaxed enough to decode the meaning of your emotional reactions about certain topics. Why do certain topics arouse the feeling of vulnerability or helplessness or defensiveness in you? Connect the dots and you will know the origin of your reactions.

I came to understand why law of attraction

junkies would be drawn to the powerful words like: *Whatever is true, whatever is noble, whatever is right, whatever is pure, whatever is lovely, whatever is admirable -- if anything is excellent or praiseworthy -- think about such things. ~ Philippians4:8 verse:*

The game you have to play as you connect the dots of your reactions, is to close that gap with the things that feel noble, admirable, excellent... and the things that feel like they are strangling life out of your emotions.

I think the reason why people resist change is because they look at the task itself and all they see is a daunting or intimidating undertaking. People are not often told that the Soul is already ingrain with ASCENDED qualities such as noble, pure, lovely, admirable... and all they have to do is relax, so as to tap into these excellent thoughts. HAPPY thoughts causes your body to behave happily while unpleasant thoughts drag your body around like a bag of wet blanket. What would you rather have with/in you as you navigate the journey of your wellbeing?

I have arrived at the place of understanding that some unpleasant thoughts may sometimes need mental surgery -- You may need to revise the meanings you are accustomed to giving the unpleasant thing or person you see in the mirror so as to notice the lovely and beautiful aspects to admire. If that strategy helps to soothe the no-so noble grip it has on you, your worthiness will shine.

This inner-work of shifting from the paradigm you've been programmed with, to a preferred state of praiseworthiness, gives you a lot freedom to do whatever floats your boat. There is not a 'right' way or set of rules to soothe your inner-being, but have fun, make it playful, comforting, exciting... because Desire always feels good when it doesn't compel, but joyfully propels you forward.

Blossoming
with ease:

In the plant kingdom, sprouting and blossoming are at different stages of growth, but still belong to the same plant. So when you are sprouting, it doesn't take away from your root – the value of your wholeness!

Every plant needs oxygen!

Breather... Relax... Breathe... Nothing can ever take away your potential to live out your wholeness. Believe... Relax... breather again... With each breathe you take, you will realize your thoughts are getting lighter and lighter and they float away as you relax in the acceptance of your wholeness.

On the other hand, thinking negative thoughts about your situation is like inviting enemies around you that you already know will misuse your energy, crush your spirit, without adding any value to your wellbeing. The company of negative thoughts in your mental environment is never to uplift you nor encourage your creative ideas to flow, but it doesn't mean that if you find yourself smothered by negativity it can't be a tool for growth.

At the worried-stage? -- Trust that all is well.

In a fearful-state? – Let fear be your fuel.

Feeling shameful? -- Remember that you're so FREE, you can choose bondage or choose to see it as an invitation to uncover the hidden meaning behind the events that caused you to feel shame.

As human on this planet, your Mind is your driver and your body is your vehicle, but your emotions make great companions on this journey of ascension because the essence of their intelligence is to offer clues that guide you and nudge to your blossoming season. Keep connecting on a deeper level with yourself by breathing and paying attention to how your emotions interact with your own thoughts. The thoughts that arouse your feelings of misery can be allowed (only by you) to go away, or stay. Or, you can chose to replace them with more uplifting thoughts and watch your reaction. You will be delighted to witness how this exercise can drive you transcend what you previously thought was your prison-limit.

Never be afraid to allow your consciousness penetrate deep areas to slay your past regrets. You already generate thoughts that can give you the boost for outstanding transformation, but without checking what is in the root of the situations that provoke particular reactions, the outcome will be shallow.

Without honoring your own core balance and harmony within, leaves an opening for provocations to push you towards eating your way out of your predicaments; which is a form of fooling around with stress. Sadly, your core desires will never vanish. They are alive in your spirit and don't die with food. Even the cells in your body know that the meatiest steak and sweetest treats can only go so far as filling up the carnal part of you.

The heart of the matter is that Truth wants to emerge from that situation and show you the way of ascension -- to leave behind the temporary baggage that your body has become accustomed to; so you can dwell in the place that compliments Freedom and Joy.

What compliments Freedom? Joy'gasm:

The enemy to your Desire is stagnation! Desire's function is to summon you to the big dreams that only you see and only you hold dear; and only you know what it would feel like to have them fulfilled. Everybody is like a unique instrument. Some people have a tensed relationship with themselves and others have a loving relationship with themselves. In order to compliment the free spirit that you are, you simply find alignment with your physical and spirit Self, by being in the state of surrender.

Surrender is like having an orgasm during a loving sexual interaction. You put yourself in a state of receptivity. It is a No-tension zone where the mind is not as stringent, thus energy flows faster, you feel fully alive in the moment, you feel very okay with losing yourself in the feeling of emotional sanctuary. You are open to the experience of having what you want and pleasure is of prime concern in that moment. *That is what I call Joy'gasm!*

We are all energy. Be conscious of how you feel in relation to what you desire to manifest. Are you approaching with surrender or are you still holding your breath hoping nothing bad happens? If you've always wanted to live a life of respectful and loving relationship, bashing your body image will keep you from experiencing love; until you release that tension-causing-energy.

If your cells are asking for relief, your commitment to release old thoughts and putting in the right thoughts will serve your cells, which, by the way, are always in communication with your mind. Your cells respond to the sense of relief in your energy that your thoughts transport. The more tension you release, naturally your body will feel the need to inhale (an expression of relief). This rush of energy from deep breathing drives more oxygen and vitality into your cells and makes it a lot easier for you to lead yourself into activities that prove you are choosing to express the idea that you are free. Own it... and enjoy your Joy'gasm anytime!

Closer & closer within range of what your soul needs:

There is always a probability that not everyone is at the point of complete certainty and clarity of owning their freedom. And that is okay. Nobody is asking you to get up one day and suddenly be perfectly aligned with the person you fully admire.

But what you can do is move one step at a time to get within range of your 'thrown of Grace' where you are presented with what's needed for your moments of weakness.

My family makes several trips throughout the year for various reasons. Whenever we are on these road trips out of town, I have noticed that on isolated parts in the countryside or in buildings that are not wired with the necessary network capabilities, carrying on a clear conversation with someone on the other end of the line is difficult. If it is an outdated network system with limited or zero reception in that area, then all we do is struggle to understand each other because the conversation keeps getting interrupted or the words don't quite sound the way we are saying them.

The difficulty is not always in speaking but even basic phone functions like sending a text. I may write the best text message but if the network signal is low, it will not send my message and that will be confirmed when I receive a "failed to send" notice. At that point, what is required of me is either I leave the environment altogether or I find a spot where the network reception is clear. It is the same with your inbuilt human "network of attributes" – when the energy of your point of attraction is low, you experience tension and resistance and at that level, you cannot fully function and expect outstanding results.

Some people say "but I know what I need to do, still can't do it"... Yes, you may have the head-knowledge about the subject, but it doesn't close the gap to bring you to the place of experiencing your True Nature (powerful, peaceful, free), because you are not connected via the appropriate channel, or our channel is blocked by a network of anger, jealousy, sadness, hurt or pain.

That's a frustrating scenario, isn't it? Especially if you know you can have easy access to your Abundance. The feeling of helplessness and frustration about your health or weight gain is an obvious sign that there is distortion in your 'network'. It is a hint that your perception of the TRUTH is misplaced, because when you know the Truth, you are armed with clarity and confidence, not helplessness.

Remember this and keep it in your memory:

YOU are Not powerless! You are Free!

YOU are never without power!

Yes, it is possible to find yourself in a situation where you want to live without feeling bad about the state of your health, but you are NOT powerless. It could be that you have forgotten how to close the gap with the holistic version of you. You may have allowed yourself to be tempted by food to feel better because you have given food an emotional power.

Your REAL power is in your Awareness; where you see yourself in relation to your Divine Source. This, to me is the missing link to healing your attachment to food.

So before you jump into the seductive industry of any diet programs, first come to terms with the fact

- where you are is where you are... don't judge or condemn yourself... you have the power to let go of the invisible mental imprison you are in.

- From where you are, you can start telling a new story -- a new story about how your life could be, how gloriously inspired you are. And if the "NEW" story is too far from your current reality, just open a different chapter to a more **believable** topic.

- You may not be able to jump from frustration to faith overnight but as you keep that hopeful spirit, destiny will bring you and faith together as mutually devoted partners on this journey.

- It is not about perfection outside but most importantly it is your inner growth that makes those hard days meaningful.

- Faith will always remind you that you are not alone, but that your path to fit and healthy is paved by Self-Love.

- The more you acknowledge the abundance within you, the more you gain more confidence to keep the faith, because you draw from the assurance that you are being guided.

- Faith will make you see the person you wish to BE, and empower you to see the possibilities rather than your mistakes.

- Be open to the richness of experiences that the journey can bring, starting NOW... Be relaxed. Be receptive.

Take five minutes to observe your reaction changing instantly.

Are you smiling?

Not yet?

Do I see a smile?

Okay I'll give you more time to SMILE.

I mean really SMILE.

Keep smiling...

Your Cells loves to see this part of you because you are being easy on yourself, freeing yourself.

It's time to stop the bullying! What some of us know about bullies is that they rush to judge, condemn, intimidate, belittle and attack the people they bully. They treat them with lack of respect and usually influence how others see the bullied individual. The relationship between the bully and the person being bullied is strained, mean and downright cruel. It is very rough.

I bet you'd say No, if I asked "Do you like bullies?" But do you know that when you are hard on yourself it is a form of bullying? If you don't like bullies, then why are you being a bully to your Body-Temple? You see the correlation between those who are labeled 'bullies' and what you do to your body when you judge, condemn, belittle and disregard her? I know a lot of women who talk about their bodies as if they are referring to the person they hate. You'd often hear something like

"Eeww you need to see my stretch marks"

"Eeww my stomach is so flabby"

"Eeww I hate my skin tone after childbirth"

"Eeww my love handles are embarrassing"

"Eeww I need to get rid of this fat"

"Eeww, eeww, eeww……."

When you have such strong negative reaction

towards something, you make it unappealing and you attract energies that affects how you treat it. See, it's not a myth that if I don't like something, hanging around what I dislike can easily provoke an unkind reaction from me, and from that negative reaction, (meaning I don't like how I feel when I interact with the thing I dislike), I will be inclined to misjudge and conclude that it is unworthy of my love and respect.

But all that brutality and bullying can stop. It can end when you switch the key to start APPRECIATING simple things about he body you were given to navigate this earth. If you're beginning to smile, feeling hopeful, stay there... That energy of anticipation is your higher Divine Source making a path in the Spirit realm; cutting off anguish, removing distress to reveal a better version of you.

~Chapter Fourteen~

Resonance & Surrender

What I have happily shared with you is what I learned from personal experiences, interacting with the Universal Mind, learning about how Universal laws govern our lives from the inside-out. However, if something doesn't resonate with your soul, you are a FREE Being; and you can exercise your freedom to skip it.

What works for me is in accordance with my beliefs, which might differ from yours. Resonance is what determines effectiveness. That said, the law of attraction, just like the irrefutable law of gravity is effectual, and freaking works!!!

I am excited for your journey ahead. I hope I have done my part is raising your awareness and helping you SEE your spirit-person with a fresh perspective. You are a glorious Goddess who deserves a life of Ease, Joy and high Energy.

It has been an adventurous ride for me too, but utmost Joy to share the "inner-game" to reveal that skinny, healthy and vivacious version of you.

You have the option of LOVING YOU. You have the option of inviting excitement into the process. I am looking forward to seeing you receive your breakthroughs and I want you to know that I am with you in Spirit, expecting your manifestations. Remember that it is only over when you quit. So be focused, and if you need my support to navigate your journey, I am available in myriad ways.

I believe in your ability to exceed your perceived limitations; so stop hiding behind an average person...

It's time to surrender any strongholds.

Time to surrender your past.

Time to surrender your guilt.

Surrender your need to prove yourself to anyone or explain to anyone your True Self. You are here because God wants to work with you to co-create your desired abundant life. You can fight it, argue, defend or ...Surrender To The Spirit In You that created the Universe: This shows how important you are - You are One with the GREAT I AM!!!

ABOUT THE AUTHOR

My name is Therra, a "Free Spirit", a wife and mother
of three(3) children, and CEO of Sakkacise; a fitness
and wellness coaching program.
My THERRA'py is the embodiment of joy, peace, fun
and many hours quietly soaking in the bathtub.
Wellness is my passion and inspiration is my gift.

*I have endured losses due to multiple miscarriages & stillbirth,
plus Diastasis Recti (abdominal split) after childbirth, so I
understand if your body has also been through some "abuse" and
how tumultuous events can ruin your focus and deplete your
energy;... But I also KNOW we all have spiritual prowess to
overcome forces that threaten our success.*

Oh dear, what a journey we're on…
Now the only thing left for me to do is to invite you
to celebrate life with me; for it is a new dawn.

It's a new day

It's a new life for meeeeeee

And I'm feeling, feeeeeeeeeeeeling, feeling

Goooooooooooood

http://www.sakkacise.com

211